T0352867

Sound Healing
for Beginners

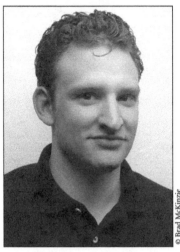

Joshua Goldman is a lifelong sound healer. His father is renowned sound healing pioneer Jonathan Goldman. From the time he was born, Joshua has been surrounded by and worked with sound as a healing modality. He was raised around numerous luminaries in the sound field. Through the years filled with workshops and teachings, Joshua has gained a deep knowledge of sound healing on both the technical and experiential levels. Joshua is passionate about spreading knowledge of sonic modalities, and he is excited to see a world where more people explore and benefit from the transformational power of sound.

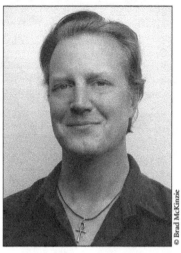

Alec W. Sims has been involved with music and sound-related pursuits his whole life. Alec was a professional musician for many years before discovering the world of sound healing. He still performs, playing guitar with various popular Colorado bands. Alec has worked with Jonathan Goldman's Healing Sounds since 1998. He has been a core staff member at the annual International Healing Sounds Intensive for eighteen years and the facilitator for the Healing Sounds Correspondence Course since 2002. During that time, he has done personal consultation sessions with hundreds of students from a wide variety of backgrounds. His harmonic overtone chanting is featured on many of Jonathan Goldman's most popular CDs, such as *Ultimate Om, The Lost Chord,* and *The Divine Name.*

For more information on the ongoing work of Joshua Goldman and Alec W. Sims, please visit www.sound-nexus.com.

Sound Healing

For Beginners

Using Vibration to Harmonize
Your Health and Wellness

Joshua Goldman
Alec W. Sims

Llewellyn Publications
Woodbury, Minnesota

First Edition
Eighth Printing, 2023

Cover art by iStockphoto.com/18452683/©agsandrew
Cover design by Ellen Lawson
Edited by Stephanie Finne
Interior art by the Llewellyn Art Department except figure on page 195 by Mary Ann Zapalac.

Llewellyn Publications is a registered trademark of Llewellyn Worldwide Ltd.

Library of Congress Cataloging-in-Publication Data
Goldman, Joshua, 1988-
  Sound healing for beginners : using vibration to harmonize your health & wellness / Joshua Goldman, Alec W. Sims. -- First edition.
      pages cm
  Includes bibliographical references.
  ISBN 978-0-7387-4536-7
  1. Vibration--Therapeutic use. 2. Mind and body. 3. Health. I. Sims, Alec W., 1966- II. Title.
  RM721.G598 2015
  615.5--dc23
                              2015007858

Llewellyn Worldwide Ltd. does not participate in, endorse, or have any authority or responsibility concerning private business transactions between our authors and the public.
  All mail addressed to the author is forwarded, but the publisher cannot, unless specifically instructed by the author, give out an address or phone number.
  Any Internet references contained in this work are current at publication time, but the publisher cannot guarantee that a specific location will continue to be maintained. Please refer to the publisher's website for links to authors' websites and other sources.

Llewellyn Publications
A Division of Llewellyn Worldwide Ltd.
2143 Wooddale Drive
Woodbury, MN 55125-2989
www.llewellyn.com

Printed in the United States of America

Thanks and Dedications

Joshua would like to thank his father, Jonathan; mother, Karen; stepmother, Andrea; his unflappable coauthor, Alec; and all his friends and family who offered him support.

Alec would like to thank his parents, William and Carol Sims, for all the love and encouragement they offered during their lifetimes and dedicates this work to their memory. Alec also thanks all of the participants of the Healing Sounds Correspondence Course for sharing their energy and sounds. Students can sometimes be the best teachers!

We would also like to thank our editor, Angela Wix, for her saintly patience and encouragement over the course of the writing of our manuscript. You are an angel!

contents

exercises

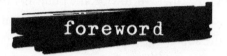

foreword

by Jonathan Goldman

Sound is one of the most amazingly important, powerful, and interesting subjects imaginable. *Sound Healing
for Beginners* will make this subject fascinating and fun. Alec
Sims and Joshua Goldman are two of the most knowledgeable and gifted writers in this field. While this is not the first
foreword I've written, this particular one has a synchronicity
that I must share with you.

I've been in this field of investigating and teaching the
uses of sound and music for healing since the early 1980s.
I'm the author of numerous books and over twenty-five CDs
that focus on the therapeutic and transformational nature
of sound. With acknowledgement of my credentials, I can
tell you that sometime in the mid-1980s, a gentleman by the

name of Carl Llewellyn Weschcke (who was the owner and chairman of Llewellyn Worldwide, the publisher of this outstanding book) and I were in negotiations about my writing a book on the subject of sound healing. I had just finished my thesis for a master's degree from Lesley University. The subject was using sound and music for healing. Carl was very interested in my turning this into a book. So was I. But other things came up and alas, that particular book with Llewellyn Worldwide never manifested.

Fast-forward to thirty years later. I received an e-mail inviting me to write a book for a company that went by the name of Llewellyn (which by now has become much larger and more prestigious than when I was first contacted but still can claim to be the world's oldest and largest metaphysical publisher). Due to prior contractual agreements with other companies with which I was engaged, I had to decline the offer. But I found it quite extraordinary that the opportunity to manifest a book for Llewellyn had occurred again—thirty years later. This time I did not give thanks and politely hang up the phone because it was not possible. Well, I couldn't anyway—it was the Internet after all and this was an e-mail. Instead, I wrote back something like: "Though I am unable to take part in such a project, I know of two people that would do an excellent job and who I would highly recommend."

Thus began the journey of this book, which may have actually had its initial start quite a long time ago in the 1980s and is now finally manifesting. I truly give thanks to the two people I recommended and who took the ball from there (or whatever euphemism you want to use to describe continuing the process set in motion from my recommendation of them).

These people are my son, Joshua Goldman, and Alec Sims, our Healing Sounds OM (which either stands for Operations Manager or something equally noteworthy since the first initials of the title spell out the sacred sound *om*). Alec has also been the director of the Healing Sounds Correspondence Course since 2002, which from experience alone makes him quite an authority on teaching people how to use sound as a healing modality, for he has now done hundreds of one-on-one private consultations with students from a wide range of backgrounds. His extraordinary harmonic overtone chanting is also featured on a number of my most popular CDs.

Of Joshua Goldman, there's little I can say other than the fact that since his inception on this planet, he's been a continued inspiration for me. In fact, the first original recording I created for Spirit Music was a sonic birthing environment titled *Dolphin Dreams* and was created for Joshua's birth. At the time, it was the first commercially released recording that featured the sounds of dolphins (as well as whales, the ocean, human heartbeat, and much more), and many still utilize it for the birthing process as well as for deep relaxation and meditation.

I don't know how many other infants, toddlers, teenagers, young adults, or even adults have been exposed to the myriad of extraordinary and different sounds that Joshua has experienced. He was playing around with crystal bowls and Tibetan bowls in the early '90s, before he had even learned to walk. I can still see him hitting the bowls with the striker he held and the glee on his face. This is just one of the many memories I have of Joshua's involvement in sonic experiences. I won't embarrass him any further with parental remembrances. The fact that he did not reject sound healing due to his upbringing (despite teen rebellion years, etc.) is an incredible testament to the fact that not only is he a gifted writer, graduating cum laude with a degree in writing, but that he has also embodied the experiences of sound with which he was brought up. I give thanks.

I remember the first time I met Alec Sims. It was at a very special workshop I gave in Boulder, Colorado, in 1996 with Lama Tashi, who was then Umzey (or Head Chant Master) of the Drepung Loseling Monastery in India. I do not recall how Tashi came to be in Boulder at the time—I do remember that we gave the workshop together in a very special "multisensory" laboratory at the University of Colorado. This was a room designed to give deaf people the ability of experiencing sound. So there were all sorts of strange and unique aspects to the room, including floors that vibrated with speakers underneath them, which allowed those in the room to feel these sounds via bone conduction. There were also colored lights that flashed on and off whenever sound occurred. It must have been quite a unique experience for those in this workshop (who, incidentally, were not hearing impaired) to feel resonance of the Tibetan "deep voice" that both Lama Tashi and I were able to create.

Alec Sims was among those in that workshop—a workshop the likes of which (to my knowledge) has never been repeated. There were a number of other extraordinary beings who also attended that workshop, including my wife, Andi. I know because I have on the wall in my office an 8 x 10 photo of the group as we chanted a Tibetan mantra that day.

This workshop could well have been a follow-up from a previous workshop. Alec and Andi would know better than me about this. Regardless, there was something quite special and precious about this workshop. Among other things, it led to some extraordinary connections and continuations with others who attended it. Some years later, Lama Tashi would come to teach at the Healing Sounds Intensive, Andi would become my wife, and Alec would become our OM.

Of all the beings I've known, Alec has always been among the most knowledgeable about sound and spirituality. We've shared many discussions on various aspects of the subject and passed books and the like back and forth with each other. He's also an exceptional guitarist, and we once performed together at a Music and Health in American Music Conference at the University of Colorado back in 2005 in a presentation called "Blues as Healer." That's also another experience that's never been recreated. At least not yet.

Alec has attended, assisted, and ultimately taught at nearly all of the Healing Sounds Intensives. Joshua began doing the same when he had reached an appropriate age to interface with adults at the event. They are like etheric brothers to each other and together have led the Boulder Toning Group for several years now.

Okay—I've introduced your writers. Now, on to the subject of sound healing. Except that you need only go to the table of contents to see the depth and clarity of information and material found within this book. It is outstanding. So rather than write on topics already found in *Sound Healing for Beginners*, I'd like to share a rather personal memory that I trust is relevant to the book and particularly to this foreword.

In the mid-1980s, I remember giving one of my first lectures at the New York Open Center, which was then considered quite an esteemed place to have a presentation. I gave information about the different principles and practices of sound healing throughout the world—for example, how many of the ancient creation myths involve sound, which is something that both our modern quantum physicists as well as the spiritual masters of old agree upon. However, I think that one of the most important concepts that I imparted is something that I've only hinted at in a number of my other books. It was actually the first thing that I started out with in this lecture. I know because somehow I was able to find those notes and they are directly in front of me. It says:

1. In order to fully research, investigate, understand, and use the power of sound and music as therapeutic tools, one would need to be a:
   a. Physician—to understand the mechanisms of the body (including chiropractic)
   b. Physicist—to understand the mechanisms of energy
   c. Psychiatrist—to understand the process of behavior
   d. Psychoacoustician—to understand the effects of sound upon the ear and the brain
   e. Audiologist—to understand the mechanism of the ear
   f. Mathematician—to understand the mathematics of music
   g. Linguist—to understand the study of language and speech

h. Neurologist—to understand the effects of sound upon the nervous system and the brain

i. Electrical engineer—to be able to build different instruments for creating and measuring sound and music

j. Philosopher—to understand concepts behind music's creation and use

k. Acupuncturist—to understand Oriental medicine, including meridians and points

l. Esoteric expert—trained in all occult and spiritual subjects

m. Psychic—able to see etheric fields, prophesize, and communicate with unseen forces

n. Magickian—to understand the uses of chants and magickal formulas

o. Healer—trained in all traditions; chakras, bioenergetics, etheric fields

p. Shaman—able to induce and travel to different states of consciousness

q. Vocalist—able to create all techniques of chanting and toning from all traditions

That was the first page of my outline for the lecture on the workshop I was about to do. I have not edited anything, but I still agree with what I wrote more than thirty years ago. I could perhaps come up with some more categories necessary for an individual to be an expert in order to become truly adept in the field of sound healing. But regardless, the major concept of this first page was to indicate to the audience I was talking to that it was literally impossible for one person in one lifetime (or perhaps many people in many lifetimes) to become adept in all these categories. Thus on one level, regardless of how long we have been in this field and at our particular area (or areas) of expertise, *we are all still beginners in sound healing.*

I thought at the time I first presented at the Open Center that in just a few years somebody would hold a device like a "tricorder" (the fictional medical analysis instrument on *Star Trek*) over someone and be able to scan and perhaps fix whatever ailed them. In medicine—at least traditional medicine—this has not happened yet. Even some of the most seemingly researched information about the therapeutic power of sound is still practically unknown. The sound work of Alfred Tomatis, MD, which has been utilized for many years in hundreds of centers working with learning disabilities, is still considered fringe. It is unlikely that if you asked your doctor about his work that he'd do anything more than scratch his head. The phenomenon of binaural beat frequencies—the ability of slightly out of tune sounds to entrain and synchronize our brain waves—is not something that most of the scientific community is aware of either. This, despite the fact that binaural beat frequencies have been used therapeutically for nearly forty years! Regrettably, most of this information has not made it into mainstream medicine.

Please note, you will encounter information about the above material in this book and more. The science of sound is surely important. However, you'll also encounter those areas of sound that focus on those sounds as an energy medicine—these include magickians (with a "k," indicating true magick and not stage magic), healers, and shamans. From my perspective, these are the approaches that really matter, for the knowledge and use of sound as an energetic healing modality has gone back many hundreds, if not thousands, of years. There's quite a bit of understanding of sound in these approaches, and it's the kind of information and experiences that Alec and Joshua will also share with you. You'll find out about the extraordinary energetics of sound and, in addition, find out about the physical-plane attributes of sound—how and why it can heal. These basic principles and practices of sound healing are mandatory for any "beginners" understanding in this subject.

Perhaps most importantly, in this book you'll gain the experience of the healing nature of sound through practice. Many years ago, when I was doing my initial research at Lesley University on sound healing, I was a virtual walking encyclopedia of sound healing. I could tell you details of multitudinous systems of sound healing—from Tibetan to ancient Greek to Native American and so on. But it was all theoretical information and not experiences I had received. Ultimately, it was not particularly practical or useful for myself nor for the teaching of others. Over the years, I have dismissed a majority of this data, replacing it with the understanding of experiences with sound that I have received. From my perspective, it is in this understanding that so much of the true healing nature of sound gets lost. If we deal simply with information and not experience, then something is missing. With sound, it is in the experience of sound that we gain true knowledge. Once you have experienced something, it is genuine and it is yours and is the real thing! This is something that Alec Sims and Joshua Goldman understand and know. And it is something they will share with you. From the effects of listening to the power of producing your own self-created sounds, they will present to you not only data on the hows and the whys of these subjects, they will also give you easy and truly profound exercises. Through such exercises, you will feel the resonance of these sounds in your own body, learning to feel the sound and to control the effect and outcome of it. This is not only important—it is life changing.

Thus, it is my great honor and privilege to present to you this beginners guide to sound healing, sharing the awareness that we are all "beginners" and that Alec Sims and Joshua Goldman are two of the best guides I know. Enjoy this marvelous journey into the world of sound. For many, it may only be a first step, but it may also be a path you will continue on for your entire life. What a blessing! I wish you sound travels!

Jonathan Goldman
Boulder, CO, 2015

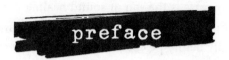

preface

Welcome to *Sound Healing for Beginners*! First of all, we'd like to thank Llewellyn Publications for this opportunity to share our thoughts and teachings with you. But, most importantly, we'd like to thank you for your interest in sound as a therapeutic and transformative modality. We have an exciting journey to share together!

Before we take the first steps, allow us to introduce ourselves. Or to introduce each other, as the case may be. We have both been deeply involved in pursuits related to music and sound for most of our lives. We owe a great debt to the work of sound healing pioneer Jonathan Goldman and his wife and partner, Andi Goldman. We would not be in a position to write this book without their love and encouragement.

Joshua Goldman was literally born into the world of sound healing. He is the son of sound healing pioneer Jonathan Goldman. Joshua was playing Tibetan and crystal bowls literally before he could walk, and he was raised in a rich environment that exposed him to leading sound healing practitioners from an early age. He led his first group chants while still barely more than a toddler. This unique upbringing contributed to a deep knowledge of the uses of sound that is beyond his years. It's one thing to learn about sound healing, but it's another to be raised with it as part of the fiber of one's being.

Alec Sims has also been involved with music and sound-related pursuits his whole life. He spent many years as a professional musician before becoming involved in the realm of sound healing. He has also been a lifelong student of many esoteric and spiritual subjects, and he always seeks to relate them to an ongoing exploration of sound. Among other things, Alec has been the facilitator of Jonathan Goldman's Healing Sounds Correspondence Course since 2002. During that time, he has done personal one-on-one consultations with hundreds of students. This direct interaction with students' personal needs and experiences has cultivated a unique understanding of the power of sound to facilitate shift and change and has contributed greatly to the perspectives offered in this book.

So that's who we are, in a nutshell. But before reading further, we ask that you now say your name out loud and offer a brief introduction as to what brought you to these pages. We always begin groups by asking people to state their name and an intention. Even though this is a book, and we're not physically present together, this simple ritual will help form a connection. For, as we will explore shortly, sound is a force that both touches the basic physical world and has influence on subtle energetic levels. Perhaps even nonlocal magickal levels! The act of making sound creates waves that literally move molecules, and thus has very real effects on the world around you. These effects are just the tip of the iceberg. As you offer your introduction, begin to feel that we are a nonlocal group, gathering together at different times and places.

Where to begin? As Jonathan Goldman notes in his gracious foreword, sound healing is a vast field. Sound work draws from a multitude of different disciplines and can be applied or adapted in many arenas. To be a fully realized sound healer would require proficiency in a wide range of skills. In spite of that, the profoundly powerful starting points can be very simple. Our approach will be to discuss sound through the lenses of several different traditions and frameworks of thought. All of these fields are heavily influenced by sound and offer many insights from which sonic techniques can be gleaned.

We apologize in advance for being somewhat selective in our choice of topics. There are many other subjects that could be discussed in the light of sound. We can only offer a few that we feel to be most significant. Similarly, we can only offer the briefest, hopefully inspirational, discussions of how sound relates to these traditions. There is always much more that could be said. In that spirit, we will also offer a recommended resources section and bibliography, which will allow you to explore the subjects we introduce even further.

Of the many filters through which sound work could be viewed, one of the most expansive models is to think of sound as a branch of energy medicine. For indeed, sound may be the "gateway" energy work modality. Everyone can hear and feel the effects of sound, whereas more specialized sensitivity and training may be required in other subtle energy modalities. Unless operating from a natural talent, the abilities to see auras, feel energy emanations with the hands, project energy as in a practice such as Reiki, etc. are typically less common than the natural ability to hear. But through working with sound and the power of one's own voice, one's sensitivities to these other forms of energy will be enhanced. And, as we will discover, there are many subtler dimensions within even the audible bandwidth of sound that will open up as we proceed. These finer aspects of sound form the bridge to higher octaves of vibrational work and, ultimately, to explorations of your own higher consciousness, which is where the master musician resides.

We live in an age where there are vast amounts of information at our fingertips. A simple search on the Internet will open immense libraries of data on any given topic. This is also true of sound. It is easy to find many different schools of thought pertaining to sound work, ranging from time-tested wisdom to various more speculative claims along the lines that a certain frequency is the frequency of "love" or that another frequency is the only truly correct pitch to be used for the tuning of instruments. We encourage such contemplations and explorations! But do not be overly quick to accept any bit of information as the final truth, and be on the lookout for claims that come from highly biased sources. In the words of the late, great esoteric philosopher Robert Anton Wilson's 22nd Law: "Certitude belongs exclusively to those who only own one encyclopedia."[1] Perhaps "to those who only consult one website" would be an appropriate amendment to this law in the current age of information.

That being said, we will also offer a lot of information and recommendations. We will first introduce some basic principles of the nature of sound and then proceed to various ways you can use sound to create shift and change in your own energy field, your states of consciousness, and ultimately, how you can broadcast these new fields of vibration out into the world for the benefit of all. Take what we offer as a starting point, for there is something in the field of sound for everyone. As you explore, you will find the particular niches that resonate most strongly with your own being.

Above and beyond the level of facts and information, there's definitely one thing we know to be true—the power of the sound current itself. Therefore, our main suggestion for how to use this book is to actually do the various sound exercises that we offer. As you enter into the realm of pure experience with sound, sound itself will become your primary teacher and source of initiation. As you resonate with sound in the energetic laboratory of your own mind, body, and spirit, new levels of insight will unfold far beyond what the printed pages or words on a computer screen can offer.

Make the time to be in sound. You will be glad you did! And, perhaps more importantly, allow for the time to be in silence after the sound. These still points can be the time

---

1. Robert Anton Wilson, *E-mail to the Universe: And Other Alterations of Consciousness* (Tempe, AZ: New Falcon, 2005), 241.

when the greatest insights will come to you. We would also suggest that you have a journal on hand to keep a record of any experiences or inspirations that may result. Allow for some time to create a record of your own unique results after each sounding exercise.

On that note—let's begin! Prepare to tune up your instrument, which in this case is the energy field of your own being.

We honor and invoke the masters of sacred sound, wherever they may be found—in all genres of music and in all spiritual traditions—and, most importantly, the master of sound within *you* who is now ready to awaken and sound forth.

In Resonance,
Joshua Goldman
Alec W. Sims
Boulder, CO, 2015
www.sound-nexus.com

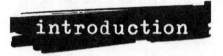

introduction

The World Is Sound

The knower of the mystery of sound
knows the mystery of the whole universe.
—HAZRAT INAYAT KHAN

Listen. What do you hear? Spend a moment taking note of any sounds that come to your attention. Now close your eyes. Take a deep slow breath, and release it fully. Take another breath, and release it slowly and completely with a slight breathy sighing sound. Pause for a moment. Now listen again. Keeping eyes closed, first direct your attention to the closest sound you perceive. The first sound may be the sound of your own breath, or if you are inside, perhaps it's something in the room with you. Now allow your attention to expand to a sound source farther away. Perhaps you are able to hear a sound in the next room, or maybe on the floor above you. Let your awareness continue to expand. Extend your consciousness beyond the boundaries of the space where you currently find yourself. What is the sound farthest away that you can hear? Listen to it. See if you can clearly visualize the source of that sound. Can you also merge with it and feel it?

After a couple moments, drift back and let your attention return to your breath. Open your eyes to return to full awareness of your current surroundings. How do you feel now? Does your energy feel different? Perhaps expanded somehow?

We live immersed in an ocean of sound. Perhaps, like fish dwelling in water, we may not always be conscious of its presence and effects. Yet it is always there, acting on us in ways ranging from the subtle to the profound. Sound is with us our entire lives. Hearing is the first sense to develop. It has been determined that hearing is active around the sixteenth week of development in the womb. Unborn babies can hear and react to sounds. Pregnant women have reported feeling the fetus move in a startled response to loud noises. Studies have even found that babies who are sung to while they're in the womb recognize the same tune when it's sung to them after they are born. And just as hearing is the first sense to develop, it's also the last one to leave us before death. We swim through currents of sound throughout our entire life journey.

The use of sound as a therapeutic modality dates back to prehistoric times when shamans chanted and drummed to heal people. In the ancient mystery schools of Egypt, Greece, India, and other centers of knowledge, the use of sound and music for healing was a highly developed sacred science. Numerous spiritual traditions honor sonic vibration as the fundamental creative force in the universe. Though the use of sound and music for healing has ancient roots, we are only now witnessing a tremendous emergence of awareness of the power of sound as a tool for transformation.

Why is sound so fascinating? Perhaps because sound is ever-present. While it's possible to cover your eyes to block out light and pinch your nose to block smell, it's not possible to completely shield yourself from sounds. The late avant-garde composer John Cage once went on a quest to experience complete silence. His journey led him to seeking out an anechoic chamber, which is a type of sensory deprivation room that filters out all external sound. He expected that the anechoic chamber would provide the culmination of his quest—that he would finally experience true silence.

Yet inside the chamber he was stunned to still hear two sounds—a low-pitched rumbling and a high-pitched drone. When he exited the chamber, he asked the assisting technician about the nature of these sounds. The assistant replied that the low sound was that of blood circulating through the body and the high sound was the nervous system in operation.

This experience triggered an epiphany for Cage. While on one level there was a failure of his initial goal to experience complete silence, it led to the more expansive revelation that sound is always with us. It is impossible to ever experience true silence!

Yet what is sound? In the most general sense, it may simply be thought of as a manifestation or expression of energy. It's simply that bandwidth of energy that we perceive primarily through the ears. Yet the experience of sound is not limited to the sense of hearing. It may also be perceived on a basic physical feeling level via skin and bone conduction. On its fundamental level, sound is a physical-plane energy form.

Its vibrations are transmitted by molecules literally bumping into one another. Our most common method of perception of sound is through the air as picked up by the ears. But, as noted, the whole body receives and resonates with sound.

Although we will focus primarily on the power of sound in the pages that follow, it quickly becomes fascinating and inspiring to consider that the range of frequency that we perceive as sound represents a relatively small slice of the full spectrum of vibrations. This bandwidth of perception we hear provides only the beginning of a sonic glimpse into the richly complex vibratory nature of reality. For example, consider a common dog whistle. We can't hear it, but when blown it produces a loud, piercing tone for a dog far above what humans experience as sound! And the limits reach much higher—dolphins can perceive frequencies over one hundred times greater than the limit of the human range. That's an astronomical increase above our level, yet to them, it's sound. It's difficult to conceive how that level of frequency would be perceived.

Thus, we begin with the foundational concept that sound is a form of energy that first expresses itself on the physical plane level. It is perceived most prominently via our sense of hearing, yet this perception may well be only the tip of the iceberg of the vibratory nature of reality. Just as hearing itself extends far beyond what we can physically hear, the principles of sound extend, at least analogously, through all the octaves of vibration. Sound may rightfully be thought of as the gateway energy modality that provides a comprehensive model offering profound insights into all others.

Sound as Energy Medicine

In recent years, there has been an explosion of books on the market offering teachings and information pertaining to a field known as energy medicine. A fundamental concept of this discipline is that energetic fields are the primary component of reality. Physical matter is a manifestation of energy. The old Newtonian paradigm of the billiard ball universe where physical matter reigns supreme is evolving, giving way to the more fluid concepts that matter is solidified energy that is subject to shift and change in response to fluctuating energetic patterns. The underlying and overlaying energetic fields surrounding a physical manifestation represent higher orders of information and reality than the often-temporary physical form.

There have been many fine works released in the energy medicine field by authors and teachers such as Donna Eden, Barbara Brennan, Richard Gerber, and many others. Their materials are highly recommended. Yet it's intriguing to note that in discussions of the more subtle manifestations of energy that typically lie outside the range of normal sensory perception, many of the ideas are expressed in terms borrowed from the world of sound. Points are made using terms such as *resonance, vibration, wavelengths, pulsation,* etc. In the introduction to her book *Energy Medicine*, Donna Eden offers a perfect perspective to form the bridge between the subtle energy nature of reality and sound:

Energy is the common medium of body, mind, and soul. Its wavelengths, rates of vibration, and patterns of pulsation form their shared vocabulary, much as the fluctuations of tone and tempo form the vocabulary of music.

The more fluent you become in sensing this shared vocab-
ulary of body, mind, and soul, the more skillfully you can
orchestrate their lifelong symphony.2

And there we have it in a nutshell! Energy manifests
in patterns of vibration. And these patterns often organize
themselves into fields and ultimately structures that can be
meaningfully compared to music, which could be conceived
of as organized sound. While these terms are often used as
metaphors in discussions of more subtle forms of energy,
when working within the bandwidth of sound they can be
experienced as direct perceptions. This experiential accessibility offers one of the most striking advantages in working
with sound! In the subtle energy realms, practitioners are
often required to develop finer levels of perception. While
such things as the ability to see auras, feel subtle energy
flows, etc., are very real, they often involve specialized training or idiosyncratic innate abilities. The distinction that provides sound with the edge is that everyone can hear and/or
feel sound. Through the study and, more importantly, the
experience of the universal principles of vibration via sound,
profound insights may be gained into all of the subtler forms
of vibration.

Another significant aspect of energy medicine is how
the consciousness of the practitioner is profoundly involved
with the effects and results. One common maxim is "energy
flows where attention goes." An energy medicine practitioner's focus of intention and attention provide major factors

---

2. Donna Eden and David Feinstein, *Energy Medicine: Balance*
   Your Body's Energies for Optimal Health, Joy, and Vitality (New
   York: Jeremy P. Tarcher/Putnam, 1998), 2.

in the outcome of any practice or procedure. Guided visualizations and focused imagination are often the main tools of energy workers. Since sound is just another type of energy, all of these techniques and methods may also be applied to working with it.

Above and beyond those approaches, sound has the powerful edge, once again. As a physical-plane energy form, sound literally moves and vibrates matter. Physical plane sound, in and of itself, is capable of shifting and changing molecules and cells. When combined with the techniques of visualization and focused consciousness taught in the schools of energy medicine, the synergistic addition of physical plane sound may well contribute the master ingredient to a fully realized energy medicine paradigm!

There is a powerfully evocative phrase in the Vedic tradition stated as *Nada Brahma*. This term is often translated as "The World is Sound." But with a bit of additional analysis, it yields more profound implications. In essence, *Nada* means "sound," and *Brahma* is a name for the creator god in the Vedic tradition. *Nada Brahma* equates the two terms. Thus, the phrase *Nada Brahma* not only implies that sound is the creator but that the creator god is sound! If this concept seems outlandish to a conventional Western mind, it's interesting to note that the same perspective is also plainly stated in the Bible:

> *In the beginning was the Word, and the Word was with God, and the Word was God.*—John 1:1

This simple verse makes a stunning statement. God not only uttered creative sound in the form of the Word, but God was the Word, and the Word was God. God is sound, even in the traditional Bible.

Although it's tempting to dismiss such theological thought forms as mere metaphor, there may well be much truth to these scriptural claims. Scientific experiments have conclusively demonstrated that sound has the power to create and shape physical form. As we will see, contemplation of sound quickly leads to profound metaphysical speculations. Furthermore, and perhaps more importantly, the direct experience of sound can open the gateway to deep mystical and spiritual realms. The essence of sound is not to be found in words on a page or in studying various theories. The experience of sound in the personal laboratory of your own mind, body, and spirit will provide the ultimate validation and value. Sound itself will be your primary teacher and source of inspiration and initiation.

In the pages that follow, we will further explore these perspectives and paths. We will first offer a fuller introduction to sound as a physical-plane energy form. We will then explore ways in which energetic fields, forms, and states can be created and shaped via sound. Then, perhaps most importantly, how form, emotional and psychological states, and ultimately reality can be shifted and changed via sound. For just as we can all hear and perceive sound, we can all also create sound, and thus become creators of the ultimate creative force! *Nada Brahma!*

Recommended Reading

Energy Medicine by Donna Eden and David Feinstein

The Healer's Manual: A Beginner's Guide to Vibrational Therapies by Ted Andrews

Quantum Healing: Exploring the Frontiers of Mind/Body Medicine by Deepak Chopra

Subtle Energy: Awakening to the Unseen Forces in Our Lives by William Gerber

Vibrational Medicine: New Choices for Healing by Richard Gerber

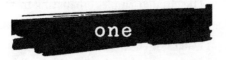

one

The Physical Energy of Sound

Music and sound are the language
and architecture of the cosmos.

—TOM KENYON

As we have already noted, sound is ever present. And as we will continue to explore, the sound that we can hear is actually only a small fraction of the ocean of vibrations that surrounds and envelops us. However, let's always remember that we are not separate from the sound; we too are producing sound from the core of our beings. So we are continually co-creating a universal web of sound. We are affected by it, but in turn our waves help blend into the symphony of the web and affect all around us. Sound forms the basis of a unified field that connects us to all of physical reality.

With that concept in mind, let's talk first about the sound we can audibly perceive. What is sound? Sound is a form of energy caused by vibration. All sound travels in waves. To visualize this concept, imagine tossing a pebble into a still pool of water. The circular ripples emanating from where the pebble lands illustrate a simple type of wave motion. The rippling effect on water is an example of one type of wave known as a mechanical or pressure wave. A mechanical wave requires a physical medium to travel through. Sound is also a mechanical/pressure wave, but one that radiates out in three dimensions from its source.

The science of acoustics is extraordinarily complex. It would require an extensive dedicated textbook to fully address the topic. Our purpose here is simply to introduce some fundamental concepts to serve as a working vocabulary to begin to delve into the practical applications of sound. In order for sound to exist, there must be three conditions present. First, a substance must have an elastic quality that will permit it to expand and contract. Second, there must be an energy or a force that will cause the substance to vibrate. And third, there must be a medium through which the resulting vibration will be carried. In other words, there must be an object that can vibrate, a force or energy that causes it to vibrate, and then a means by which these vibrations can travel. In the example above, the impact of the pebble on the surface of the pond causes the elastic substance of water to vibrate, the surrounding water is the medium through which the vibration travels, and the ripples are the sound.

The Measurement of Sound

Sound is measured in cycles per second, which could be conceived of as the number of waves that manifest from crest to crest in one second. In the case of audible sound traveling through the air, the source of the sound creates waves in air molecules in much the same fashion as the pebble tossed into the pond ripples the surface of the water. A cycle per second is simply another way of describing the number of waves that reach your ear in one second.

The common technical term for the number of cycles per second of sound is *hertz*, abbreviated Hz, which we will use for the remainder of this book. The number of hertz of a sound is also known as the sound's frequency. Humans can generally hear between about 20 and 20,000 Hz. Low sounds, or sounds with a low number of hertz, have longer, slower-moving waveforms that are subjectively experienced as very deep or bass sounds. High sounds travel in faster, shorter wavelengths. To give some perceptual context, the lowest note that you can hit on a standard tuned piano will produce a frequency that vibrates at 27.5 Hz. The highest note on the keyboard vibrates at 4,186 Hz. The average conversational adult male voice has a fundamental frequency of between 120 and 150 Hz, and the average adult female voice has a fundamental frequency between 210 and 240 Hz. The high end of a female soprano's singing range extends slightly above 1,000 Hz.

Sounds below 16 Hz or above 20,000 Hz are considered beyond the standard range of human hearing. These inaudible sounds are known as either subsonic (or infrasound) or ultrasonic, respectively. Different individuals, or course, have different "normal" ranges of hearing and, indeed, there are large percentages of the population who cannot hear above 10,000 Hz. When we are younger, our hearing range is larger, and as we age it is common to lose the higher aspects of the range. At the time of this writing, Joshua can hear at a maximum of around 16,000 Hz, which he perceives as a very high faint whining buzz. As the sounds grow faster in frequency, he loses the audible perception of them altogether, but as we know the sounds are still present and still touching and affecting him.

Different animals are capable of not only hearing frequencies much higher or lower than those within the human range of hearing, but some can also produce them. Sounds in the range of 20–100,000 Hz are commonly used for communication and navigation by bats, dolphins, and other species. These frequencies are inaudible to us, but for them they are heard as sound. So it is useful to begin thinking of sound as an energy form that expands well beyond our bandwidth of hearing. This phenomenon will be important to recall as we proceed to discuss the more subtle energetics of sound.

Another important measurement for physical sound is amplitude. Amplitude refers to the height of the sound wave, which contributes to the perception of its intensity and volume. The larger the amplitude, the louder the sound will be. The loudness of sounds is measured on a logarithmic scale using units know as decibels, abbreviated as dB. To give you a general frame of reference, here are some decibel levels of common sounds:

- The sound of normal breathing registers at 10 dB.
- A whisper increases to about 30 dB.
- Normal conversation takes place at roughly 50–65 dB.
- A dishwasher and vacuum cleaner measure at 70–75 dB.

- A car horn measures at 110 dB.
- The threshold of pain begins at 120 dB. Prolonged exposure to amplitudes of around 90 dB and above may result in hearing damage.
- Examples of sounds above 120 dB include jet engines and shotgun blasts.

As we have seen, sound waves are created by vibrations. Everything in existence is vibrating, even if it seems perfectly still, because on a subatomic level there are moving particles. Therefore, if an object is vibrating, it is putting out a sound, whether or not it falls into our audible bandwidth. This means all things have a natural vibratory rate known as their resonant frequency. We can think of it as the fundamental tone of the object.

To imagine this phenomenon, think of a wine glass. Gently tapping on the glass produces a clear bell-like tone. This tone is the resonant frequency of the glass. Every object has a resonant frequency, whether or not we can audibly hear it. This book has a resonant frequency as do the individual pages. The chair you may be sitting on has a resonant frequency, as does every other object within your current surroundings. In fact, you have a resonant frequency. All your organs, bones, tissues, and parts of the body have their own separate resonant frequency. Together they make up a composite frequency that contributes to your own personal resonant frequency.

Yet as we have noted, nothing exists in pure isolation. Everything affects and is affected by the vibrations of a multitude of other entities and phenomena in the vast web of vibrations. There are two important principles that interact with and affect objects. These principles are resonance and entrainment.

Resonance

The term *resonance* includes several different subcategories. How the phenomenon of resonance manifests depends on the complexity of the vibrating body or substance. The first category is called free resonance. This aspect of resonance relates to a simple object's basic resonant frequency. Through the principle of resonance, the vibrations of one body can reach out and set off vibrations in another body via an exact match of the object's natural resonant frequency.

Let's think of the glass again. We've all seen or heard of singers breaking a glass with their voice. First the singer matches the resonant frequency of the glass with her voice, which sets it into vibration. As the singer proceeds to put more powerful sound energy, or amplitude, into the glass, the vibrations ultimately become too intense for its structure, causing it to shatter.

A simple experiment with tuning forks could serve to provide a demonstration of free resonance. For example, if one were to hold a tuning fork of a certain frequency, say 100 Hz, and then strike another tuning fork of 100 Hz and bring it near the first tuning fork, the first tuning fork will also resonate and sound. The matching frequency of the second fork stirs the first into vibration via a sympathetic transfer of energy. This effect can also be multiplied. One could assemble an array of ten 100 Hz tuning forks, strike one, and they will all sound. However, if you were to change the active sound source and strike a new tuning fork of say 120 Hz, the standing 100 Hz forks will not sound.

The next evolution of resonance is known as sympathetic resonance. In this case, the principle is expanded beyond an exact match of frequencies to frequencies that are related in a harmonic fashion. We will discuss harmonics in more detail shortly, but for now it is sufficient to note that the most significant harmonics result from doubling a basic frequency. For example, if you begin with a frequency of 100 Hz, the pitches at 200 Hz, 400 Hz, 800 Hz, and so on will all be strongly related.

Sympathetic resonance can be most easily demonstrated on a piano. When you step on the damper pedal of a piano, all of the strings within the piano body are free to sound. In this mode, any note played will cause all of the other strings of the same pitch to also resonate. For example, one could play a low C note and all of the other C strings would also sound. All of these C notes are related to each other via the doubling of frequency effect, and thus they all will sound according to the principle of sympathetic resonance.

The third and most complex category of resonance is known as forced resonance. To understand this principle, we must consider the evolving complexity of vibrating bodies. Resonating substances can be divided into two general categories. Certain simple substances, such as tuning forks, are only able to resonate at their natural frequency. Yet other substances that are more elastic in nature have the ability to resonate at a variety of frequencies. Examples of the most elastic substances are air, water, some woods, the human body, and indeed the earth itself! Therefore forced resonance describes the capability of more complex bodies to vibrate and react to multiple frequencies. This principle opens up an exciting world of possibilities! Substances are not limited to vibrating at one single, fixed frequency, but are more fluid and subject to shift and change. This fluidity provides one of the most significant foundations for the power of sound healing—frequencies can shift and change in an ever-evolving dance.

Entrainment

The phenomenon of entrainment is the second major principle by which bodies can influence each other's frequencies. In a sense, entrainment could be considered a subcategory of resonance. But it does seem to have a more active element. Entrainment is when the powerful vibrations of one object will actually change the vibrations of another object, causing this second object to lock in step or synchronize with the first. This synchronization is a phenomenon of nature that seems to have to do with the conservation of energy. Entrainment happens all the time in the world around us, whether it is between humans, such as two people coming into step with each other walking down the street or a group of dancers pulsating with the beat of a band, or between inanimate objects, such as metronomes set to different rates coming into perfect unity.

The classic demonstration of entrainment is attributed to the Dutch physicist Christiaan Huygens in the seventeenth century. Huygens was a contemporary of Isaac Newton and was also the inventor of the grandfather-style pendulum clock. He once arranged a room full of these clocks of various sizes. He proceeded to go around the room starting the pendulums of the clocks in motion at different times. When he left the room, the pendulums were all swinging at different individual rhythms. When he returned the next day, he was surprised to find that all of the pendulums were locked in step with the largest of these clocks.

Like the pendulums of Huygens's clocks, our internal biological rhythms are also subject to entrainment. Our heart rate, breathing rate, and brain wave activity all entrain with each other in a powerful feedback loop. Our heartbeats will entrain with our breath. As many know, deep breathing slows down the heart rate, which in turn calms the nervous system, which results in slowing down the predominant brain wave rhythms. When the breathing rate slows, the heart rate slows in turn, which helps to relieve the fight-or-flight response of the sympathetic nervous system.

The sympathetic nervous system is responsible for creating our stress response. It increases our heart rate, which is fantastic for running from a predator but is not necessarily helpful in most modern stressful situations. Just as deep, slow breathing is helpful in relieving the stress response, making sound can have the same positive effect. If you want to experience this immediately, simply take a few deep, long breaths. By slowing down your respiration in this manner, you are also slowing down your heart rate and brain waves. Conversely, when you slow down your brain waves, you also slow down your heart rate and respiration.

Sounds Are Complex

Now that we have considered the elementary ways vibrating bodies can affect one another, let's add another crucial element in understanding the nature of sound—sounds are complex. While it's a valuable convenience to discuss a single basic resonant frequency of an object, in reality there are no naturally occurring single frequencies. Even seemingly simple tones such as lone notes played on an instrument are actually composites of multiple different frequencies. A pure singular frequency, known as a sine wave, does not appear in nature. To conceive of a sine wave sound, recall the tone played during an emergency broadcast system announcement. That stark, harsh tone is very close to a pure sine wave. To begin to understand the multilayered intricacies of sound, we must consider the phenomenon of harmonics.

Harmonics, or overtones, occur whenever sound is created. All sounds that are produced are mixtures of component harmonics that contribute to a rich spectrum of sound. The most basic manifestation of harmonics occurs as whole number multiples of the fundamental. For example, if the basic starting fundamental frequency is 100 Hz, the next overtone will be vibrating twice as fast, at 200 Hz. From there, the next overtone vibrates three times as fast, at 300 Hz, the fourth at 400 Hz, and so on.

In the everyday experience of sound, harmonics are responsible for the tone color of different instruments and our voices. The musical term for this phenomenon is timbre. Just as you can hold a prism to white light and refract the different colors of the rainbow, harmonics could be thought of as providing the colors of sound. They are always there, but it often takes a certain extra bit of perceptual training before they can be distinguished from the primary fundamental.

To begin to appreciate this fact, think of the difference between the tones of various musical instruments. In a classic experiment performed years ago by Bell Laboratories, recordings of different instruments playing the same pitch were processed through an electronic filter that removed all of the harmonics. After the filtering was complete, all of the instruments sounded the same! Without the richness provided by the harmonics, a piano sounded identical to the violin, which was indistinguishable from a French horn, which sounded just like a trumpet. They all sounded like that stark sine wave tone of the emergency broadcast signal—lifeless and flat. The complex structure of harmonics is what adds life and vibrancy to sound.

The discovery of the phenomenon of harmonics is typically attributed to Pythagoras, a Greek philosopher who lived circa 570–500 BCE. Although it is highly likely that this knowledge stems back to ancient Egypt and perhaps even older sources. Pythagoras was responsible for many important contributions to the developing sciences of mathematics, astronomy, and geometry. But for our purposes here, he is also recognized as one of the founding fathers in the field of acoustics. Pythagoras was highly acclaimed as a mystic. His work delved into the esoteric mysteries of music and mathematics, which continue to have relevance to the understanding of sound and music as therapeutic and transformative modalities today.

Pythagoras is credited with uttering the thought-provoking aphorism "study the monochord and you will understand the secrets of the universe." A monochord is simply a single vibrating string. The seemingly basic phenomenon of a single vibrating string provides the best gateway to begin to understand the nature of harmonics. And, as we shall see, the simple string is really not so simple; it may well offer a profoundly intricate model of the vibratory complexity of all physical reality!

The Harmonic Series on a Single String

The sound produced by a string begins with a simple overall motion. The vibration of the complete string over its full length sounds the basic fundamental frequency. For simplicity, we'll consider a string vibrating at 100 Hz. The string motion could be pictured as:

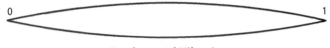

Fundamental Vibration

But this tone is just the beginning. Pythagoras determined that the string also vibrates in many different segments. If one divides the string in two, the result is two halves sounding at twice the original frequency, or 200 Hz:

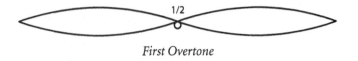

First Overtone

This progression continues through all whole number divisions of the string. A division by three produces three sections vibrating at 300 Hz:

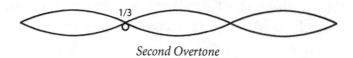

Second Overtone

This progression would conceptually proceed to infinity, but for practical purposes, human perception seems to be limited to distinguishing only about sixteen divisions. Here is a diagram of the next four:

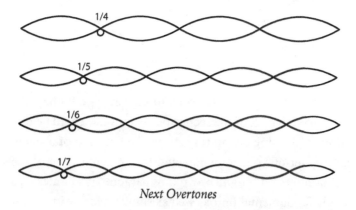

Next Overtones

These divisions of the string provide the model for the harmonic series. Exactly as demonstrated on the string, harmonics vibrate in whole number multiples of the basic fundamental frequency. They are omnipresent in all natural sounds, which is why describing anything in terms of a single simple frequency only provides the tip of the iceberg in depicting the complexity of its full vibratory reality.

But in further consideration of the string, Pythagoras noted that the string actually vibrates in all of these segments simultaneously. So in order to form an accurate model of the motion of the string, all of the diagrams above would need to be superimposed on top of each other in a composite figure:

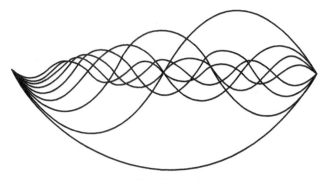

String Composite

This image perhaps begins to convey why Pythagoras concluded that all of the secrets of the universe could be discovered in a single vibrating string. The motion of a string is a mysterious phenomenon, and the contemplation of the string offers a thought-provoking paradox. It vibrates as a single fundamental unit as well as simultaneously in a multitude of conceptually infinite subdivisions. As one travels into the sound, a universe of intricate sounds within sounds unfolds. Ultimately this multitude of component frequency divisions may well extend down into the quantum realm of pure energy.

At this point we reach a crossroads. As we have seen, even the simplest sounds are comprised of a rich dance of finely interwoven waveforms. If the simple vibrating string has such nuances, imagine how much more complex and subtle things get as we move into the realm of more elaborate three-dimensional structures. And then compound the issue even further when considering the intricacies of living organisms.

Holistic Sound

In recent years, there has been a great deal of research into the therapeutic effects of various frequencies. This type of work is all very valuable and fascinating. We applaud it wholeheartedly and look forward to seeing how these avenues of exploration will continue to evolve. However, this type of research is still in its infancy. For even though sound and music have been used therapeutically since the dawn of mankind, the precise theories, methodologies, and procedures have yet to be fully investigated, validated, and quantified.

The greatest breakthroughs have been demonstrated in the application of specific pure tones, such as ultrasound projected into the body. Yet these therapies are often still largely operating within the framework of the more mechanistic allopathic medical model. While profound results have sometimes been achieved, these methods could perhaps be best termed as frequency-based therapy. As we have seen, the holistic phenomenon of sound is expansively richer than just single simple frequencies, and the effects of sound may extend far beyond simplistic frequency analysis.

Rather than being a limitation or criticism, we feel that this perspective opens the gateway to an inspiring realm of possibilities that is enforced and validated by cutting-edge progressive science. The insights provided from the realm of quantum mechanics demonstrate how the observations, expectations, and beliefs of researchers affect physical matter and concretely influence the results of experiments. If the vibrational roots of sound do indeed stretch down into the quantum realm of pure energy, then the crossroads of interaction between energetic vibration, consciousness, and matter may be the most important realm to consider when placing sound in the context of energy medicine work, as sound may well provide the most profound bridge between consciousness and the physical manifestation of matter. We will explore various considerations of this endlessly creative realm of possibility in the remainder of this book.

Recommended Reading

The Healing Forces of Music: History, Theory and Practice by Randall McClellan

Healing Sounds: The Power of Harmonics by Jonathan Goldman

Musician's Acoustics by Scott Parker and Jamison A. Smith

This Is Your Brain on Music: The Science of a Human Obsession by Daniel J. Levitin

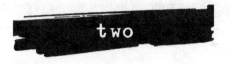

two

Listening

The eye takes a person into the world.
The ear brings the world into a human being.

—LORENZ OKEN

L et us now take our first steps into the world of sound, which is easy! The good news is—you're already there! As we noted a few pages ago, we're already surrounded by waves of sound and have always been. The first gateway into exploring the vastly intricate world of sound is to begin where you already are. This fact is true of many heroic journeys. The journey of one thousand miles begins with a single step...or one listen.

As we shall soon discover, however, there are many levels of listening, which can evolve to ever more refined states of awareness and consciousness.

Although we have noted that the perception of sound is truly a holistic full-body phenomenon, we will begin with the focus on the audible sound as perceived by the ear. On the surface, the ear appears to be a simple organ, yet it contains a vast universe of complexities beyond the visible surface structure.

Physical Hearing

On a basic anatomical level, the ear can be divided into three sections: the outer, middle, and inner ear. The outer ear consists of the visible exterior ear, the auditory (ear) canal, and the eardrum. Sound waves are funneled by the exterior skin down the auditory canal and vibrate the eardrum. The three small bones of the middle ear, known as the hammer, anvil, and stirrup, transfer the vibration from the eardrum to the cochlea, or inner ear. Within the cochlea, fluid set into motion by the middle ear moves the basilar membrane, causing tiny hairs known as cilia to bend. This sends electrochemical impulses that our brain translates into our incredibly rich perception of sound.

This process is incredibly intricate and would take half a textbook to describe in full detail; however, the punch line is that the ear performs an incredible transduction of physical energy into the world of subtle energetic perception. On a physiological level, the ear performs the mysterious alchemy of bridging the physical and the energetic realms.

Although the ear is our primary organ of hearing, its roles extend far beyond. The ear is the starting point for pathways that reach down to the deepest levels of our physiology and govern many of our core functions. Of equal or greater importance to hearing, the ear is the primary regulator of our sense of balance. In terms of our neurological wiring, nearly all cranial nerves lead to the ear. To list a few, the ear is closely associated with the optic nerve, the oculomotor nerve (which controls eyeball and eyelid movement), and the nerves that govern the musculature of the neck. The ear is also intimately tied in with the vagus nerve, the longest nerve in the body extending from the brain stem to the abdomen.

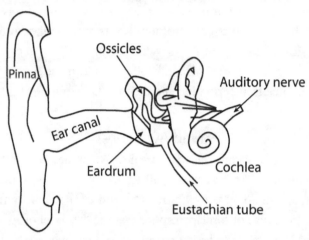

Ear Diagram

The vagus is integrally connected with many primary functions. Most interestingly, the vagus nerve governs the larynx, which is the physical structure that plays the most fundamental role in vocalization. Thus, listening is intimately interrelated to creating vocal sounds. What we are able to hear synergistically influences the sounds we are able to create.

The vagus nerve also connects to the bronchi, the heart, and the gastrointestinal tract. This opens the gateway to insights regarding how sound and the ear play crucial roles in affecting vision, breathing, heart rate, digestion, and many other bodily functions. When one considers its far-reaching connections, the ear could truly be thought of as our master sensory organ!

So as we can see, the sounds we perceive have far-reaching effects throughout our nervous system and physiology. The anatomy involved is much more complex and intricate than what we have sketched, but noting the extensive connections of the ear serves to open the gateway to considerations of how hearing can trigger profound shifts and changes in our physical and energetic states. Which brings us back to one of the major themes of this book—how you can use sound for intentional transformation and therapeutic effects.

Sound Awareness

The journey begins where you are now. An orchestra of sound is playing all around you at all times, and the component instruments of this orchestra shift and change constantly. Let this dance of sonic perceptions be the first level of sound play! The simple decision to focus on sound can be a stepping stone to powerful meditations, for sound has a unique ability to bring you into the present moment and into greater attunement with your own physical being and presence.

The foundation for shift and change first begins with an awareness of what is in the now. If you are inside during the still of night, the ambience may consist of subtle sounds that are overshadowed during the bustle of the day. Step outside in the morning and you will hear the sounds of the world coming to life. Different times of day will yield different movements in the symphony of sound, as will changes in environment. In the city you may hear the rumble of traffic or sirens in the distance, while in the country you might hear the breeze rustling through leaves, birds chirping, or the peaceful melody of a babbling brook.

As you tune in to the sounds around you, begin to take note of any associations they trigger for you. Do certain sounds make you feel anxious or alert? Do others make you feel comfortable, safe, and at greater peace? This reactionary introspection can yield intriguing insights into your own psychology. For those of you who would like to take a deeper excursion into this type of exploration, we recommend *The Listening Book* by W. A. Mathieu, which contains a wealth of guidance for experiencing the rich treasures of experience that can be triggered by pure listening.

After taking note of any associations environmental sounds may trigger for you, try to take it a step further. Begin to dissociate from any personal reactions and begin to perceive the sounds as pure energy. Performing this shift may well open you to expanded new levels of experience and relationship with the sounds. W. A. Mathieu outlines this process:

> There is a hearing meditation that has two parts: first you unlisten; then you listen. Unlistening means clearing sounds from their associations, which are often unconscious. Make them conscious. If bird song means replenishment, know that. If the sound of traffic makes you shrivel inside, know that. ... Maybe it is not possible to strip all the layers of meaning away from sounds, but at least you can evaporate the surface thoughts. The more completely you do this, the more sound will reveal its true nature. The act of identifying your psychological response is a ticket to an

even deeper response. ... Once you have identified an asso-
ciation, shoo it away. Choose to listen past it into the world
of sensual vibration. ... When thinking calms down, even a
little bit, sound wakes up.3

This type of creative disassociation can be another powerful step toward experiencing sound as pure energy. As the
boundaries of personal associations dissolve, the realm of
wider energetic potential begins to open.

The Mysticism of Sound

As the sense of energetic expansion begins to evolve, the next
step into a more mystical relationship with sound begins
with consideration of the intimate connections it forms. The
renowned deaf percussionist Evelyn Glennie has noted that
"hearing is a form of touch."[4] This statement is both a beautiful metaphor and a deep truth. Given the physical nature
of sonic energy, all of these sounds we have mentioned, no
matter how distant, are literally touching you. It's an interesting and fun concept.

Listen again to a sound in your environment. Take a
moment and focus on that sound. Imagine how as the source
of the sound vibrates it sends out energetic pressure waves
that expand until they reach you. They reach your ears and
make you consciously aware of the sound source, but they
also touch you all over via skin and bone conduction. In a

---

3. W. A. Mathieu, *The Listening Book: Discovering Your Own*
   Music (Boston: Shambhala, 1991), 22.
4. *Touch the Sound: A Sound Journey with Evelyn Glennie*, directed
   by Thomas Riedelsheimer (2004; New York: Filmquadrat, 2004),
   DVD.

very real way, you are experiencing the sound on a full-body level. And when we consider the physiological connections discussed above, we realize that these sounds are also touching us on deep internal levels. As we have noted, considering the intricate nerve pathways governed by the ear, skin is not a boundary. The energy of sound penetrates far beyond surface level physical touch.

This realization fuels the sense of mystical connectedness inspired by sound. It's a two-way street—we are not only capable of listening to the orchestra, but we are part of it ourselves! Reverse the thoughts in the previous paragraph and imagine the sounds emanating from your body and reaching back and touching the source of sound near you. These sounds are affecting one another. Resonance and entrainment are synergistic two-way streets that form a palpable form of contact between you and the object. Now remember that just because we cannot hear something does not mean the sound is not there. Let us take a step back from imagining the sonic relationship between you and the object you hear and realize that the same relationship exists between you and everything around you.

As we will discuss in more depth in the section on vocal toning, this synergistic connection is part of why it is so important to experiment with shifting your own internal resonances thoroughly before working with anyone else. An extremely complex sonic relationship exists between you and everything around you. This relationship affects you in both subtle and profound ways. It is easy to understand how a loud, sudden sound such as a thunderclap affects you deeply, altering your nervous system and changing your internal resonances. It is not so easy to understand how a sound you cannot even hear affects you. However, just because something is very small, almost beyond notice, does not mean that it cannot have great effect. So if we are constantly surrounded by inaudible frequencies that affect us, why don't we notice them? Well, simply put, it could be because we are just used to them. We were born into this world of frequency and our bodies and fields naturally compensate for the sonic immersion.

It's also possible that these subtle energetics may require an additional refinement of awareness. Just as professional musicians spend time working to develop their sense of pitch recognition, there may well be some additional training required to fully perceive these finer vibrations. But it's also possible that these perceptions are already there, just slightly out of the average current conscious awareness.

Subtle Energy Fields of Sound

To the skeptical minded, this degree of perception may seem difficult, or perhaps ridiculous, at first, but a new perspective may come from an experiment conducted by the renowned composer R. Murray Schafer.[5] Among his many achievements, Dr. Schafer was a pioneer in the field of acoustic ecology, which is the study of the sonic connections and relationships between living beings and their environment.

In one phase of his research, Dr. Schafer was involved in a quest to determine the frequency of the primordial sound. In two different groups he was leading, one conducted in the

---

5. R. Murray Schafer, *The Soundscape: Our Sonic Environment and the Tuning of the World* (Rochester, VT: Destiny Books, 1993).

United States and the other in the United Kingdom, he asked the participants to go into a state of meditation and try to tune in to what they perceived as the universal primordial sound. He then asked them to report on what they heard. People in the United States commonly heard a very low note in the range of the musical pitch B-natural. In the United Kingdom, the participants heard a note that was the equivalent of about a G-sharp.

Interestingly enough, in the United States, our electricity runs off of a current that produces a hum at about 60 cycles per second. The power grid in the United Kingdom produces a hum that vibrates at 50 cycles a second. If you were to transform those sounds into notes, you'd find that 60 cycles a second is in the range of a B, while 50 cycles a second comes very close to a G-sharp.

Is it possible that the participants in these two classes were sonically tapping into the electric current of the different countries? It seems so, and thus here is an intriguing example of people seemingly able to perceive a largely inaudible energetic field and translate it into a sound. The fact that the pervasive electric current was mistaken for the primordial tone of creation may well have some alarming implications, but it's still a thought-provoking demonstration of our ability to perceive and relate to subtle fields, which may be a common experience.

Can you recall a time when the power went off in your home and everything just *seemed* more silent? Part of this effect may well be due to various electric devices and appliances turning off. Those sounds are ever present and typically tuned out of conscious awareness. Yet there is also a different feeling during power outages. Everything feels quieter without the pervasive vibration of the typically omnipresent electromagnetic field of the household current. What other fields may the receiving apparatus of the nervous system be capable of perceiving? Perhaps quite a lot! Numerous studies into phenomena such as remote viewing and psychic perception seem to indicate the profound potential of expanded awareness. The fine-tuning of perceptions in the realm of sound can enhance your sensitivity of subtler levels of energy and higher octaves of vibration.

Music

The next step beyond the realm of pure sounds is to consider the phenomenon of music. Music plays a major role in many people's lives, and in the modern era of recording, music is seemingly everywhere. It's rare to step into any public place without some kind of music being present. Yet what is music? The definition of music has been debated by philosophers, creators, and composers for centuries. The oldest etymology traces the term back to the Greek word for "Muse," which reflects an interesting insight into how music has perennially been a source of inspiration. On the most basic level, to borrow the term originally coined by modernist composer Edgard Varèse, music can be conceived of as "organized sound." Yet, depending on a wide variety of individual perspectives, there will always be great debate on what sort of sounds are "musical" or not. Regardless of personal tastes, music generally tends to have communicative and expressive elements. Music could be most meaningfully thought of as a type of language that is intended to communicate or evoke moods, emotions, thoughts, and impressions to the listener. The purposes of music can run a wide gamut from idle background noise to entertainment to grander scale inspirations such as fueling cultural movements and, perhaps on the highest level, to a type of spiritual experience or communion.

To return to the theme of personal empowerment, music can be a powerful consciously selected tool for shift and change. On the most basic level, many people use music to shift their moods, and everyone has the ability to intentionally select music to suit the needs of any given moment. On one of its most primal levels, music inspires emotion. This direct experience is vastly more profound than any academic definitions of music. The ultimate power resides in the effects triggered via the listener's direct relationship to the pure sounds. This fact is true in all realms of sound-related work, as we will explore in more depth in chapter 5.

Learning how to use music listening in consciously selected and directed ways is the first and most accessible foundation for understanding the therapeutic uses of sound. Without any particular training, everyone can relate to the experience of strong emotional reactions tied to music. Can you think of a song that always makes you happy? Perhaps you can think of one that makes you sad? Are there memories tied to these certain songs for you? Maybe there are songs tied to your first kiss, a memorable summer, or a slow dance at your high school prom. Anytime you listen to music and it elicits emotion, it is an example of sound causing frequency change. At least metaphorically, emotions could be conceived of as having frequencies, much like everything else.

While it would perhaps be overly simplistic to think of emotions having frequencies that can be measured in hertz, emotions could be thought of as patterns of energy and vibration that affect one's state of being and perceptions. An emotion may have its basis in a certain feeling or flow of sensations in the body, but the psychological label one puts on such sensations is typically the deciding factor on whether one experiences a "positive" or a "negative" state. Just as one can shift and change the interpretations one attaches to the perceived vibrations of physical sound, one can also transmute the relationship with the root physiological source of emotional vibrations.

Perhaps the greatest lesson to be gleaned from sound work is fluidity. We are not fixed state "things" or static objects. The essence of our being consists of fluid processes of continually shifting patterns of energy and vibration. These patterns can shift and change, and, as we will continue to explore, sound vibrations can be employed as powerful catalysts for these shifts. Since music is one of the most accessible manifestations of organized sound, once we become consciously aware of the power of music to shift and change our frequencies, we can use it in deliberate, intentional ways. Take note of the internal shifts that happen when you listen to different types of music. Also take note if you seek out different types of music based on your current feelings. Is there a certain song that always picks you up when you're feeling down? Or do you listen to music that's in resonance with your mood?

All music can have therapeutic effects. There is no music or sound that is inherently good or bad. The setting will always play a major role in the effect of a given piece of music. For example, if one desires to go to sleep, some relaxing classical music or soothing New Age music may be good choices. Yet if one were driving full speed down a highway, more energized rock music would likely be more appropriate. Music should be selected that will boost the desired results in a particular situation. Most "healing" music is specifically composed to elicit the relaxation response and gentle meditation states. However, those conditions are not always the ideal goals. There is no objective perfect "healing" music without considering the time, place, and specific needs of the individual.

The therapeutic effects of music largely derive from the energetics of its particular genre. These energetics can often be analyzed in terms of the five elements of fire, water, air, earth, and ether. We will examine these energy classifications in more detail in chapter 6. But one can go a long way making choices based on one's own intuitive and emotional reactions to a piece of music. Simply think of the energy state you would like to enhance in the moment. For example, fast, driving rhythms will tend to boost energy and excitement. Slow, flowing rhythms will tend to relax and slow the nervous system.

In addition to the initial energetic effect of a particular genre, the intentionality and emotionality that a performer puts on the music can play a major role. For example, many older people consider hip-hop and rap as examples of harsh, even harmful music. There are undeniably many examples of rap that convey anger and negativity. But, as with most styles of music, the medium itself is inherently neutral.

The devices at work in rap and hip-hop are simply examples of some of the most primal singing forms. In essence, they consist of metered, rhyming language with drumbeats. The fusion of words and rhythm dates back to the most ancient bardic traditions. Rap and hip-hop could simply be viewed as modern urban manifestations of these compositional forms. What most people take offense to are the lyrics, which are the most apparent surface layer expression. However, there are many rap and hip-hop musicians with positive lyrics, messages, and intentions, such as the performer MC Yogi, whose work features songs containing sacred mantras from the Vedic tradition. Many people find MC Yogi's music to be inspiring and uplifting, which is a far cry from the angry, darker vibe conveyed by certain other types of rap. The energy of the performer's creative intent transmutes the end result into a completely different plateau of expression, even though the sound of the beats and rhythms is very similar.

On a wider scale, sometimes the appreciation of music simply shifts from generation to generation. Remember that when Elvis Presley first appeared his music raised so much controversy that it might have been considered a dark and corruptive force. The same charge was leveled at the early Beatles' music. Now in retrospect Elvis seems so tame as to be almost wholesome, and the best of the Beatles is some of the most loving music ever created.

Hearing vs. Listening

Although up until now we have been using the terms "listening" and "hearing" interchangeably, it's useful to draw a distinction between the two concepts. This clarification opens the gateway to bringing in more conscious control. Hearing could be viewed as the passive basic perceptual activity through which sound vibrations are received through the ear and perceived by the brain. But listening is more powerfully conceived as an active experience that begins to bring the conscious focus of the listener and the energies of imagination and intention into play.

The distinction between passive hearing and active listening was first noted and championed by the French physician Alfred Tomatis. Although Tomatis's primary practice was as an ear, nose, and throat specialist, his expansive work basically laid the theoretical foundation for the evolving field of sound therapy. Tomatis was responsible for groundbreaking new perspectives on hearing and increased recognition of the ear's profound depth of functionality. Many of the physiological facts listed above were first documented by Tomatis. In fact, he has been hailed as the "Einstein" of the ear, and, indeed, his work embodies a depth of innovation on par with psychology pioneers Sigmund Freud and Carl Jung.

But Tomatis was far from being a mere theoretician and researcher. The work that he began in the 1940s is still being practiced in active Tomatis Centers today. The application of his therapies has been responsible for remarkably effective treatments for learning disabilities, autism, depression, chronic fatigue, and immune system disorders, as well as a wide array of other personal enhancement and performance-related benefits.

How have these results been achieved? The core of Tomatis's treatment method involves a program of focused listening intended to expand one's sense of hearing. Among other approaches, Tomatis practitioners use a device called the Electronic Ear, which filters sounds in a special way in order to retrain the ear and return a full range of frequency perception. The therapies stem from the key element of Tomatis's philosophy, which is that sound is an energy form that charges the brain and nervous system. Thus, any deficiencies in the perception of certain bandwidths of frequency can result in various disorders on both the physiological and psychological levels. A full exploration of the intricacies of Tomatis's work is beyond the scope of this book. To find out more, read his book *The Conscious Ear: My Life of Transformation through Listening*. Tomatis's work provides the unshakable foundation for the value of listening as a therapeutic and transformative practice.

Sound Is an Energetic Nutrient

One noteworthy case study that brings this claim to life involves Tomatis's work with a community of Benedictine monks. This account also lends support to the health benefits of chanting and toning. The classic story, which was first chronicled by Tim Wilson in an interview with Tomatis called "Chant: The Healing Power of Voice and Ear," offers a beautiful example of how sonic nutrition can charge and enhance practical life activities.[6]

Tomatis's involvement with the monks took place shortly after the enactment of the Second Vatican Council in 1962. This council proclaimed many changes to church-related practices in an attempt to put the institution more

---

6. Tim Wilson, "Chant: The Healing Power of Voice and Ear," in *Music: Physician for Times to Come: An Anthology*, edited by Don Campbell (Wheaton, IL: Quest Books, 1991), 11.

in sync with the modern world. As a result, the abbot of a certain Benedictine monastery in France decided to make various changes to the workings of the monks under his guidance. Prior to Vatican II, the monks in this particular abbey would typically chant in Latin for six to eight hours per day. The abbot came to believe that the chanting no longer served a constructive purpose and eliminated it from the daily schedule.

In the days and weeks following this decision, the monks gradually found themselves becoming more and more tired. As more time passed, their condition continued to deteriorate into states of severe chronic fatigue and depression. With growing concern over these conditions, various health professionals were employed to help rejuvenate the population of the monastery.

The first doctor called in decided that the monks needed more sleep, but this prescription only succeeded in making them more listless—a result which is not surprising. When one feels tired and depressed, an excessive amount of extra sleep often exacerbates the feeling of tiredness.

The next physician determined that the poor physical and emotional states were due to nutritional problems. It was obvious to this doctor that the monks, who were basically vegetarians, needed more meat, so the monks changed their diet to a protein-rich "meat and potato" meal plan. The obvious oversight in this second theory was the fact that Benedictine monks had been vegetarians since the founding of their order in the fifth century. The vegetarian diet had a long history of supporting their rigorous lifestyle. After the shift to a "meat and potato" menu failed to improve their condition, Alfred Tomatis was finally called in.

It was obvious to Tomatis that the problem did not stem from nutritional deficiencies or lack of sleep, but rather due to sound. He began working with these monks, helping them to reawaken their ears and also immediately reinstating the practice of daily chanting. Within six months, the monks were able to return to their normal vigorous lifestyle. Tomatis's successful treatment clearly proved that both the actual practice of chanting and the immersion in sound during the chant sessions provided essential energetic fuel for the monks. When the chanting was taken away, the monks suffered. When it was reintroduced, they returned to their former vibrancy.

This case study is worthy of continued contemplation as we continue to explore the energy-enhancing effects of sound. Hearing is much more than just a passive perception of sensations from the external world. Sound is an energetic nutrient that stimulates and enhances the entire energy system. The continued evolution and refinement of listening yields profound benefits for both physical and emotional well-being. And these benefits are further enhanced as you proceed into more actively engaged forms of sound work.

Recommended Reading

The Conscious Ear: My Life of Transformation through Listening by Alfred Tomatis

Healing at the Speed of Sound: How What We Hear Transforms Our Brains and Our Lives by Don G. Campbell and Alex Doman

The Listening Book: Discovering Your Own Music by W. A. Mathieu

Musicophilia: Tales of Music and the Brain by Oliver Sacks

A Natural History of the Senses by Diane Ackerman

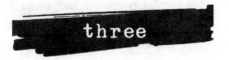

three

Conscious Listening

Let us be silent, that we may hear the whispers of the gods.
—RALPH WALDO EMERSON

In the previous pages, we have introduced some listening practices as catalysts for frequency shifts on emotional and energetic levels. We would now like to introduce yet another subtle shift and consider the interplay between listening, hearing, and altered states of consciousness.

As we have noted, we are continually immersed in an ocean of sound. Many times one does not have full control over surrounding sounds. As a result, there is often a tendency to place judgments on aspects of the sonic environment we find ourselves in. We place labels on sounds as being pleasant or unpleasant, and we often add the judgmental label of "noise" to certain vibrations.

Does a sound need to be pleasing to be therapeutic? On one level it is very helpful, because if the sound is pleasant it contributes to the state of relaxation and restful balance that is ideal for healing. But we should not dismiss the potential good of any sound just because it is initially unsettling or strange. Sometimes unusual sounds can have positive effects. For example, some people find the deep, low chanting of Tibetan monks to be very strange to the point of being off-putting or even frightening.

The Tibetan chanting known as the deep voice is certainly a very positive sound, perhaps one of the most powerful and resonant that the human voice can produce. So how do we explain this dissonance perceived by some people? Well, partially it can be attributed to a lack of familiarity. There is often an acquirement phase that people go through when first encountering something outside their cultural comfort zone. Also, the Tibetan deep voice has been used frequently in film and mass media in conjunction with images of spooky or supernatural occurrences, which creates a connection in the viewer's mind between the sound and something unsettling.

It's advisable to not automatically dismiss the healing potential of a sound because you find it initially strange. Much like the Tibetan deep voice, there are many healing sounds that initially seem unusual to the Western ear.

Sound vs. Noise

The judgment of certain sounds as noise is completely understandable (and not always inappropriate). Yet it's worth noting that if desired, we can transform our relationship to such initially unpleasant sounds with a shift in consciousness. If we can begin to listen to the myriad noises around us and hear them first as "wanted sound" (as opposed to "unwanted sound"), it may then be possible to perceive them simply as pure vibrations, and then ultimately as being "musical." This level of listening affords a much deeper level of perception than merely "hearing." Though this technique may require some practice, it can provide the foundation for forms of sonic meditation that can lead the reader into untold worlds of altered consciousness.

There are many possible benefits to this type of practice. The first practical application can relate to the basic issue of sound health. We owe awareness of this type of sonic transmutation to John Beaulieu, who is one of the most important pioneers in the sound healing field. Among many other things, Beaulieu's teachings offer keys to how to transform any sound into an aspect of the sacred sound current and to then ride that sound current to different levels of reality. We will return to this higher aspect of listening shortly. But the foundation for this higher level of practice is first provided by the concept of transforming "noise" into pure sound.

Noise Pollution

The phenomenon of noise pollution is a great detriment to the health of us all. Studies have shown how populations living near high noise pollution areas, such as airports, train stations, or truck routes, typically display dramatically higher incidences of stress-related illnesses such as heart disease and cancer. This is a grave problem that merits serious attention in our society. Much more consideration must be given to the sonic environments we construct for ourselves, where and how we choose to build dwellings, and what sort of sound sources are allowed to operate within close range of our homes.

We must begin by addressing the problem from the situation as it exists now. How does one escape the influence of potentially harmful sounds? One obvious solution for people living near high noise pollution areas would be to move. However, this luxury is not always possible. In fact, frequently it isn't an option. The fact of the matter is that many of us live near stress-producing sonic influences that are simply unavoidable. It is often impossible to avoid some kind of negatively intrusive sound source, especially in urban areas.

Of course, there are several other practical solutions to sonic pollution that we must consider before we brave the depths of changing our listening habits. The first could be to wear earplugs. Although our bodies will still be exposed to these frequencies, the sonic buffer of earplugs will block a significant portion of the sound from entering our ears and our brains. However, the wearing of earplugs poses some drawbacks. Earplugs would also unfortunately block out the things we want to hear, such as the telephone ringing or the voice of someone we are trying to carry on a conversation with. Nevertheless, like simply removing oneself from a noise-polluted environment, it is a possible solution.

Another solution is that of sonic masking, which basically involves attempting to cover up an irritating sound with a pleasant sound. For example, if a leaf blower is roaring outside your window, simply turn up your stereo and drown it out with something you like. This, essentially, is sonic masking. It is also likely the reason why half the population in major cities seems to be wearing headphones and listening to some form of music while out on the streets (or in their homes if the external sound is really loud). One problem with this approach is that sometimes what they're listening to on the headphones may not be a significant improvement sonically.

Exposure to high decibel levels, no matter what the source, can stimulate stress in the form of the "fight or flight" response. It is conceivable that people using sound masking may run the risk of being affected adversely by what they're using to mask. Of course, as with earplugs, such sonic masking not only makes conversation difficult and blocks out any other potential desirable sounds in your environment, it still doesn't stop those unwanted sounds from entering your body and electromagnetic field.

Sonic Transmutation

If such certain sounds in our environment are unavoidable, then rather than trying to block them out or mask them, the best solution may lie in striving to change our relationship and reactions to them. A powerful solution for dealing with sonic pollution involves the conscious transformation of noise into pure sound and then potentially into music.

Is this approach easy? Like many new practices, it may not be in the beginning. But is it effective? Yes! In spite of the initial challenge, it is probably the best solution to dealing with sonic challenges. Skillful use of this technique offers an added bonus above and beyond possible health benefits—it also provides the additional possibility of beginning to open your consciousness to levels of reality that you may never have dreamed existed.

The essence of the technique lies in the metaphor of the flexible stalk of wheat that bends with the strong wind as opposed to the rigid stalk that breaks. This same principle is true with sound. By opening ourselves up to different levels of sound, we can resonate and bend with the sound as opposed to fighting it and ultimately allowing it to have some adverse reaction on us emotionally, mentally, or physically. The real danger may not lie in the sound itself, but in the strain that results from our resistance to it.

Active Engagement with Noise

How does one transmute "noise" in a beneficial way? The answer lies first in expanding our understanding of what noise is. As our consciousness and awareness of sound evolves, we can begin to perceive different sounds as being pure sound rather than noise. In a way, we do this all the time. For example, when you were a child, perhaps you hated one form of music, but as you got older and became more educated to this music or heard it enough, you began to get accustomed to it, maybe even like it.

Toning or making sounds along with "noises" can provide a first step in this process of transformation. This practice facilitates a shift into a more active relationship with an "unwanted" sound rather than merely being a passive "victim" of your sonic environment. For example, if you have a refrigerator making sounds that bother you, try humming along with its vibrations. Pretty soon, you may discover a whole symphony of sounds inherent in that humming, and what once was a noise is now something you can live with and perhaps learn from. When you start sounding in harmony with a noise, all of a sudden, you become part of that "noise." As you become harmoniously united with the source of the vibration, it becomes harder to reject it as something unwanted.

This same principle is true with other noises, from car horns to motors to fire engine sirens. If we can make sounds—usually the same sounds as we are hearing—we can transform them from being unwanted hazardous noise to something else. In doing so another valuable phenomenon occurs. By sounding with the noise, we are able to release adverse vibrational patterns that can become stored in our body as tension that could potentially lead to imbalance and disease. The next time a car horn honks at you and you find yourself tensing up, imitate the sound with your own voice and honk back at the car. You'll be amazed at how quickly the tension disappears from your body. By vocally releasing these sounds, you keep them from becoming trapped within your body and energy field, which could potentially form blocks that may become hazardous to your health.

Consciously Shifted Listening

If sounding with a noise is a bit too difficult at first, begin by first trying to listen to the noise. Take a deep breath, relax, and really listen to it on a deep level. Imagine that you are completely fluid and porous and that the sound simply flows through you without hitting any points of tension or resistance. As you enter into this deeper state of resonance, close your eyes and go into the noise. Allow yourself to perceive it as a pure vibration, free of all associations. Also become aware of the sounds within the sounds. For, as we have noted, in reality there are no single frequency sounds in nature. Every sound is composed of a tapestry of harmonic overtones. As one begins to become aware of the overtones, rich new dimensions of sonic experience begin to open up. Begin listening for these subtle sonic layers, and you may find an unexpected symphony in the sounds you once thought to be mere noise.

This next level of listening opens the gateway toward transforming the physical plane reality of the sound into something else. What that "something else" may be depends upon you and your ability to open and expand your consciousness. Consider the example of the refrigerator again. Next time you listen to your refrigerator, listen not only for the overtones within the sound, but begin to imagine you are really listening to the sound of a rolling *om*, which is honored as the primordial creative sound of the universe in the Vedic tradition. If you are able to listen to the sound of the refrigerator and hear not merely the noise from a machine, you may next be able to transmute it into perceiving the music of the device. As the next step beyond that, perhaps you will soon be able to hear the pure vibration as being a room full of monks chanting a divine name or sacred mantra. Therefore, if you listen to your refrigerator humming at 60 cycles a second, you may be on the pathway to perceiving the primordial tone of the universe.

In order to develop this level of skill with sonic transmutation, it may be useful to begin with various machines and sound sources that produce white noise. "White noise" is a name given to any sound that essentially contains all sound frequencies in a unified blend. The hiss of a radio tuned between two stations and the sound of ocean waves crashing on the beach are good examples of white noise. On a side note, why it is called *white noise* as opposed to *white sound* may give us an indication of our awareness of the ability to transform noise into sound. Listening to pure white noise can be a good starting point. As you listen to white noise, you may find that it becomes like a sort of sonic Rorschach blot that will begin to evoke free-form associations and aspects of your consciousness. The next step, as suggested in the quote from *The Listening Book* in the last chapter, is to let those associations go, freeing the mind to flow on the waves of pure vibration.

In his book *Music and Sound in the Healing Arts*, John Beaulieu shares some advice on how to accomplish this goal:

> *The key to conscious listening is flexibility. Through listening, we have the ability to seek out and enter sound. When we freely resonate with sound(s) we enter into and become the sound. We are viewing the world through the sound and learn that sounds do not explain themselves; sounds reveal themselves. There are as many revelations as there are sounds and combinations of sounds, but we have to be flexible and free to move through the various realities that sounds create.7*

What Beaulieu is talking about could well open the gateway to spontaneous sonic mystical experiences to be cultivated via skillful shifts in the energy of your attention and intention. To take the first steps on this path, try the following experiment.

----

7. John Beaulieu, *Music and Sound in the Healing Arts: An Energy Approach* (Barrytown, NY: Station Hill Press, 1987), 15.

Exercise: Conscious Listening

Close your eyes and imagine you are lying on the beach on a hot summer day, listening to the sound of the ocean. Most people will find that to be quite a pleasant image. And the sound of the ocean? Just that sound alone is enough to transport us to a place of quiet and serenity. Most people find the sound of the ocean quite therapeutic, as the gentle, flowing rhythms lower brain waves and reduce respiration and heart rate. This is no doubt one of the reasons for the popularity of various environmental recordings that feature the sounds of the ocean.

The crashing sounds of waves and surf are simply a natural example of white noise. They are a full-frequency sonic spectrum that we enjoy largely because we have attached pleasant associations to them.

We have established that the sound of the ocean creates beneficial responses within our being. But above and beyond the physical reaction, when we hear the sound of the ocean, we usually use our imagination to travel to some part of our psyche that relates to the ocean sound. We are not just hearing the ocean; we are actually traveling on the sound of the ocean into the realm of imagination.

This is that next level of listening. While it may be a bit more difficult to perform with the roar of a jet plane than with an ocean, it involves the same principle. For both the ocean sound and that jet plane sound are essentially just white noise that could ultimately be perceived as sonically equivalent from the highest perspective. The ability to open up our consciousness and listen more deeply opens the gateway to perceiving them as manifestations of different degrees of the universal sound energy current. This higher level of listening allows for the profound transformation of sound.

Journeying on Sound

The last level of intentionalized listening involves one further step of cultivated imagination. To recap, we may first listen to the sound of that white noise and transform it into the sound of the ocean. Then, through the power of our imaginations, we may travel with that sound to a time and a place when we have been at the ocean. The final evolution in the process is to learn to travel on the sound so that you actually become the ocean.

By working with our imagination, we allow ourselves the opportunity to learn to travel on sound. By continuing with this, we are actually able to tap into the morphogenetic fields created by the sound, traveling to the creative source of the sound. In essence, we are becoming one with the sound.

This same level of listening could occur if we opened our consciousness enough with the refrigerator hum and traveled not just to a group of people chanting *om*, but actually traveled with the sound still deeper, until we became the *om* ourselves and went to whatever level of reality that *om* originated from. Which in this case would be the source of all creation itself.

This deepest level of listening is called the *shabda*, or sound current, in the Vedic tradition. It is considered by many to be the highest form of meditation, a powerful technique for altering consciousness and traveling to higher realms of being. You may have already experienced this more refined level of listening but simply not known how to describe it. Perhaps you thought it was merely your imagination, which of course it was, since without use of imagination such sonic traveling is not possible. In addition, you were most probably traveling on the sound current and becoming one with the sound. This sort of experience can certainly happen easily and spontaneously, but to fully develop the skill could take much additional practice. However, rich rewards can be in store for those of you who desire to undertake this journey.

The Power of Silence

Virtually any sound can be used to travel on the sound current. Nevertheless, it may be useful to initially start with either listening to simple white noise or to a particular sacred sound such as the *om* or by listening to silence.

Silence? How can one travel on the sound of silence? As we have noted, in reality, it is impossible to truly experience silence (i.e., a state completely devoid of sound). Recall the experience of John Cage noted in the early pages of this book. Cage entered a space that he expected to be free of sound, and yet sound was nevertheless discernible. The internal sounds of his own body were inescapable. Therefore, silence could be reduced to the inner sounds that are within us all. Some of the most profound journeys outward may begin by first turning within.

It has been suggested in various mystical traditions that the internal universe is as vast as the external one. Thus, the internal current of subtle silent sound may well provide one of the most potent vehicles for expansive resonant communion with the cosmos, the higher self, and the sacred. Allowing yourself time for silent meditation and assimilation can be the most valuable part of any sound practice. For it is during this time of stillness after the external physical sound has ended that the energetic resonance of your sounds will continue to echo for maximum effect.

Conscious Listening Exercises

To hopefully help bring the ideas of the following pages to further life in the realm of your own direct experience, we would like to suggest the following exercises as a two-stage sonic initiation. We will begin with an experience of your own inner sounds. We will then proceed to enhanced awareness of your external sonic environment. May these meditations serve to initiate more profound contact with the sound current!

Exercise: Internal Sound

Here is an exercise that you might try to get in touch with your inner sounds. First, find a place that is as quiet as you can find. Once you have some experience with this practice, you can perform this exercise anywhere, but to start, a place of quiet is recommended.

First, block your ears with your fingers or earplugs and begin to listen to the sounds within your body. You will hear your heartbeat and your breath and perhaps the blood circulating throughout your body. As you become quieter and more focused, you may even begin to tune in to more subtle sounds, such as the frequencies created by your brain waves.

Remember, your body and the sounds of your body are sacred. The ancients viewed the human body as a temple, and the sounds inside this temple are most certainly sacred. They may in fact be the most sacred sounds that are directly available to all who choose to go within and listen.

Next, begin to tune in to the sounds in the fashion discussed earlier in this section. As you open up to a new vista of imagination and possibility, your heartbeat may become the primordial sound of the Earth Mother or your respiration may become the ebb and flow of the life force of the creator. Tap into these sounds and let your imagination flow with them. Travel freely on the sound current with these sounds.

Like the mantras mentioned above, remember that the pulses of your breath and heart have morphogenetic fields that have been resonating for millennia. As you focus on these sounds, you can tune in to the sounds of every heartbeat or every breath that has ever sounded since the beginning of life. Travel on these sacred sounds to their source and experience that source. As you do, you will realize one of the great spiritual truths of all time—that you and the source (the Creator, God, or whatever name you wish to use) are one.

Interestingly enough, the Bible echoes one of the major tenets of sound current philosophy: "In the beginning was the Word." The Word was "I am." This "I am" principle is found in virtually every spiritual tradition. The universal knowledge and understanding of the unity between the macrocosm and microcosm and the link between heaven and earth has been summarized in the Hermetic maxim "as above, so below." This simply stated yet extremely sophisticated awareness of the relationship of self to the Creator can be directly experienced through the act of listening to the sounds within your own inner temple.

After the conclusion of this exercise, if it serves you to do so, you may wish to spend a period of time journaling. Record any notes about your experience. Jot down any insights, spontaneous thoughts, or inspirations that may come to you immediately afterward.

Exercise: External Sound

For maximum effect, it is recommended that you perform this exercise on a different day than you performed the previous exercise. As you gain experience, you may combine the exercises we offer in an extended session, but for now enjoy them as separate experiences.

As before, find a relatively quiet place where you will not be disturbed. Sit comfortably in a chair or perhaps in a relaxed meditation posture. Look around and observe the different components in the space you find yourself in, however you may perceive them. Now close your eyes. Begin to take full, deep breaths in a slow, even rhythm. Focus your awareness on your breath and particularly on the sounds associated with breathing. Listen to the flow of your inhale and exhale for a few minutes.

Next, allow your attention to shift and expand outward. Keep your eyes closed, and instead of using your eyes and your sense of sight to receive, encode, and explore information from the outside world, use your ears and your sense of hearing. Is there a difference? Become aware of all the subtle nuances of sound that may be occurring. Do you hear your refrigerator humming or the clock ticking? Is there a dog barking in your neighborhood? Do you hear a neighbor's television or perhaps their lawn mower?

Be as still as you can. Let your breath become very gentle. The quieter you become, the more conscious you will be of the myriad number of different sounds in your environment. The more you focus upon these sounds and become aware of them, the more this awareness will change the information you receive about your environment and your world. As you practice this exercise, slowly begin to shift your focus of awareness from the sounds nearest you to the sounds farthest away. What's the closest sound to you? What can you hear in the very distance? Are you able to visualize or feel the energy of whatever it is you are hearing?

As you practice this form of deep listening, become aware of any changes that may occur with your consciousness through this exercise. For example, do you feel different as you tune in to the more distant sounds versus the sound sources close by? You may even wish to pause slightly between both the inhale and exhale.

Does your sensitivity to sounds become enhanced during these still points?

Now, bring your focus of sonic awareness back to the sounds of the space you are sitting in. Allow your focus to return to the sounds of your breath. After a few more minutes, open your eyes again.

Take note of any differences you may notice after returning from your meditation. Even though you have returned to "normal" consciousness, is your awareness of your environment somehow different than before? Is it perhaps expanded in some way?

If it serves you to do so, spend some time journaling about your experience and the aftermath. Take note of how these seemingly simple shifts in awareness can trigger powerful altered states. We will consider the next steps into this realm of how sound can be used as a more active tool to shift states of consciousness in the next chapter.

Recommended Reading

The Ringing Sound: An Introduction to the Sound Current by Eric Gustafson

The Third Ear: On Listening to the World by Joachim Ernst Berendt

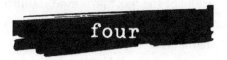

Shifting Consciousness with Sound

The Realm of the Shamanic Practitioner

> *People ask me, "How do you know if somebody's a shaman?"*
> *I say, "It's simple. Do they journey to other worlds?*
> *And do they perform miracles?"*
>
> —MICHAEL HARNER

In the last chapter, we offered various methods for changing one's relationship with sound via intentional shifts in consciousness. We would now like to consider the inverse perspective—how sound may be employed to induce shifts in consciousness. These two approaches may be used on an ongoing basis in a powerful synergy. The roots of these techniques may be found in the ancient shamanic traditions.

Shamanism may be the root source for all spiritual traditions as well as the original form of energy medicine practice. The explosion of energy medicine teachings that are available to us today may well be a reawakening of systems of knowledge that were only known to an initiated minority in past eras. Many of the most profound traditions of shamanism employ deep use of sound techniques, which makes the study of shamanism of great value to both sound workers and students of energy medicine in general. The essence of shamanism is not theory or "faith" based; it can only be understood via an experiential, direct knowing.

What Is Shamanism?

In many cultures throughout the history of humankind, there have been traditions involving special individuals who have possessed remarkable abilities to communicate and interact with the natural and spirit worlds. However, the practices that these figures engaged in often seemed alien and strange to early European observers. As anthropological perspectives became more sophisticated and compassionate, the term *shaman* came into common usage. The word *shaman* derives from the language of the Tungus people of Siberia. The appreciation of these practitioners has evolved significantly in recent years, and the word has been adopted to apply to a wide variety of practitioners from non-Western cultures who play very special roles as emissaries between humanity and the spiritual realms.

Appreciation for the profundity of the shamanic tradition has increased greatly in recent years. The popular series of books by Carlos Castaneda, which began with the 1968 publication of *The Teachings of Don Juan: A Yaqui Way of Knowledge*, awakened the imagination of a whole generation to the magical world of shamanic practice. His writings continue to inspire many seekers today.

Although the truthfulness of certain aspects of Castaneda's accounts has been called into question, his work still reflects a deep familiarity with the worlds of shamanic practice that could only have come from an in-depth study of at least some accurate source material. Nonetheless, the popularity of Castaneda's books opened the door for Michael Harner, who could be viewed as the true pioneer who introduced the shamanic worldview in a way that was accessible to Western readers.

In his book *The Way of the Shaman*, Harner defines a shaman as a man or a woman who enters an altered state of consciousness to contact and utilize an ordinarily hidden reality in order to acquire knowledge and power and to help other people. Shamanism may be understood as an ancient system of healing involving techniques for entering into and interpreting the depths of the psyche encountered during journeys to other worlds. Shamans also often have guardian spirits, such as power animals or totems, from which much of their power and knowledge is derived. This phenomenon may be the root for contemporary practices in various intuitive and energy work fields relating to getting in touch with one's "higher self" or "guides."

Shamans are found in numerous cultures throughout the world. The Hopi of the United States, the Jibaro of South America, the !Kung bushmen of southern Africa, the Iglulik of Hudson Bay, the Wiradjeri of the Australian Aborigine, the Chukchi of Siberia, and the Tibetan Bon, to name just a few, all incorporated shamanic figures in their society. Depending on the culture, the roles played by the shaman vary widely, ranging from healer, priest, intermediary between the living and the dead, and messenger between the animal and spirit worlds.

As the ancient and sacred traditions of shamanism have gained much wider recognition, the knowledge of the healing techniques has become widespread in the holistic health communities. This evolution is well deserved, for shamanism is probably the most time-tested system of using the spirit, mind, and heart for healing. Shamanic healers still work in contemporary societies side by side with modern medicine.

Shamanic practice has stood the test of time simply because the methods work. In the traditional societies, the shaman is typically judged on the basis of practical, demonstrable results. Effective cures or results are either achieved or they are not. There is no faith-based element. The practice of shamanism is a method, not a religion. It also coexists with organized religions in many cultures. In light of this widespread efficacy and adaptability, it comes as no surprise that many alternative therapists are now studying shamanic techniques to aid and enhance their own work in our modern culture.

But it is worth noting that true shamans often underwent arduous trials and periods of training. So it is imperative that the term be employed with the proper respect. The shamanic tradition, besides being very ancient, is also very sacred. Most often, a shaman was an exceptionally gifted being, who either through illness, psychic experiences, or some other measure, gained the ability to travel to the underworlds and spirit realms. Shamanic power was often acquired at the expense of much hardship and learning. The initiatory journeys often posed very real risks to the apprentice shaman's sanity, if not his life. If fact, many obeyed a calling to the shamanic path that was not willfully chosen.

The shamanic tradition is an initiatory tradition, whether these initiations were the result of external vision quests or internal journeys to other planes of consciousness. One did not all of a sudden wake up one day and say, "I think I'll be a shaman!" Shamanic abilities were earned through years of work and experience in order to open the consciousness to levels of reality that are not normally viewed, let alone explored in heroic depth. The ability of the mind to travel to worlds within worlds and to reach out to realms beyond—all the while understanding these other realities in such a skillful way as to return to accomplish practical results on the physical plane—is an awesome feat.

Therefore we believe it is important to make a distinction between a "true" shaman who has been initiated within the framework of long-standing tradition and a shamanic practitioner. In recent years, there has been an explosion of information relating to shamanic practices, and many Westerners may very well have received very authentic training, but it is crucial to avoid using the term *shaman* too freely in such a way that inadvertently conveys disrespect to the source traditions. It would be a bit like referring to oneself as a PhD without actually passing the necessary examinations or adopting the title of MD without doing the hard work required to obtain a medical degree.

It's likely that only a select few people will be in a position and have the resources to make the complete commitment necessary to become a true shaman, yet many of the insights and teachings from these traditions can be applied and adapted in beneficial ways to enhance various healing, meditative, and self-development practices. A person who does so could perhaps be better referred to as a shamanic practitioner or as someone who employs techniques gleaned from shamanic traditions, but is not necessarily a shaman per se. Therefore, when we refer to shamanic practices, please understand that we mean to relate them to a shamanic practitioner who uses sound techniques to enhance and empower his or her work.

Exploring Altered States of Consciousness

Shamanic practices come in many forms, but there are some universal common elements. After years of extensive research, Mircea Eliade, in his authoritative book *Shamanism: Archaic Techniques of Ecstasy*, concluded that shamanism underlies all the other spiritual traditions on the planet, and that the most distinctive feature of shamanism—but by no means the only one—was the journey to other worlds in an altered state of consciousness.[8] This perspective has been echoed by later writers. According to Dr. Jeanne Achterberg in *Imagery in Healing: Shamanism and Modern Medicine*, "Shamanic practice involves the ability to move in and out of a special state of consciousness."[9] This special state of mind is sometimes also referred to as a mystical state, a trance state, or a non-ordinary reality. Michael Harner makes basically the same statement more poetically saying, "The shaman moves between realities,

---

8. Mircea Eliade, *Shamanism: Archaic Techniques of Ecstasy* (Princeton, NJ: Princeton University Press, 1951).

9. Jeanne Achterberg, *Imagery in Healing: Shamanism and Modern Medicine* (Boston: Shambhala, 1985), 13.

a magical athlete of states of consciousness engaged in mythic feats. The shaman is a middle man between ordinary reality and non-ordinary reality."[10]

Carlos Castaneda first coined the term *non-ordinary reality*. His first few books are filled with strange and sometimes terrifying accounts of his initiations into these realms. Many of Castaneda's experiences were triggered by the ingestion of psychotropic plants, which has unfortunately led to a common misconception that psychedelic substances are required for shamanic practice. While it is true that certain shamanic initiations and experiences were enhanced or induced through the use of mind-altering plants, the use of these herbs, plants, and other natural substances is not a prerequisite for shamanic work.

Indeed, based on his studies of global shamanic traditions, Harner notes that shamans use psychedelic drugs to change their state of consciousness in a minority of the cultures where shamanic traditions thrive. Many other methods were also employed to push the apprentice shaman beyond ordinary limits such as periods of prolonged fasting, various sensory deprivation practices, or vision quests that required spending many days in the wilderness. In all cases, the end was the same—to expand the shaman's boundaries in order to gain the ability to communicate with and journey to the spirit world.

We will keep in mind that the ability to shift one's consciousness opens a major gateway to being able to accomplish healings of all varieties. While methods of initiation may

---

10. Michael J. Harner, *The Way of the Shaman* (San Francisco: Harper & Row, 1990), 55.

vary, all shamanic traditions make powerful use of music and sound. Drumming, singing, and chanting are some of the most powerful methods for shifting one's consciousness and physical and energetic states.

Sound in Shamanism

As we have already noted, shamanism is thought to be the oldest form of healing known to mankind. In shamanism, the shaman communicates with the spirit world in order to do his or her work. The use of chants, songs, and drumming is the universal common denominator in all shamanic systems.

The Voice

We will begin our consideration of the uses of sound in traditional shamanism with the voice. The human voice is the most healing and mystical of all instruments and may be the most powerful instrument for invoking spirits and traveling to the spirit realms. There are, in fact, shamanic cultures such as the Wayana of Guyana that rely almost exclusively on the use of chanting and toning to do their work. While they may occasionally employ a rattle, drum, or some other instrument, the main magical sound is the voice. The sounds of nature, spirits, and various energy forms are all created solely through the power of the voice.

Many times shamanic chants or songs have been gifted to the shaman from encounters with power animals and spirits or obtained through meditations and dreams. In his fascinating book *Drumming at the Edge of Magic*, Mickey

Hart shares some examples of the ubiquitous power of song in shamanic experience such as:

> *It fascinated me that one of the first and most crucial gifts of the spirit world to the shaman is a song. A !Kung woman, describing this transmission, told anthropologist Lorna Marshall that God had stood next to her and repeated the song over and over again until she could sing it perfectly. Another woman shaman, an Alaskan, told the explorer Knud Rasmussen that "songs were born in stillness while all endeavored to think of nothing but beautiful things. Then they take shape in the minds of men and rise up like bubbles from the depths of the sea, bubbles seeking the air in order to burst. This is how sacred songs are made." 11*

Although shamanic songs often had supernatural inspiration, they sometimes also consist of known words and melodies passed from one shaman to another for particular purposes, such as chasing away a disease or removing a particular affliction. But it is worth noting that in many cases, the chants utilized by shamans often sound like wordless strings of phonemes with no literal translation in ordinary speech. Among other possibilities, such chanting may serve to bypass the left brain to tune in the shaman to more intuitive states of mind that open the gateway for the shamanic trance.

However, it is not necessary to rely on academic information! Through the practice of certain types of toning and

---

11. Mickey Hart and Jay Stevens, *Drumming at the Edge of Magic: A Journey into the Spirit of Percussion* (San Francisco, CA: Harper San Francisco, 1990), 169.

chanting, you can form your own direct relationship with the sound current and be in a position to enjoy firsthand similar types of initiations and experiences reported by traditional shamans. We will introduce the foundation for such techniques in later chapters, but we will first consider here some of the other easily accessible sonic tools that may also be useful in facilitating shifts in consciousness via sound.

The Drum

While the voice may ultimately be the most powerful and intimate means of altering consciousness, the drum is one of the most common and profound external instruments. Drumming is an ancient practice. The remains of drums have been uncovered in Paleolithic archaeological sites. These early drums have been found in close vicinity to the mysterious cave paintings, which are generally assumed to have served magical purposes. While the exact function of these drums may never be fully known, it is highly likely that, similar to the cave art, they were employed in ceremonial or ritualistic ways.

One of the conclusions that the renowned scholar Joseph Campbell drew from his surveys of world mythology was that shamans were the first artists, the first musicians, and the first storytellers. And since the drum is the core instrument in most varieties of shamanism, it is reasonable to speculate that shamans were the first drummers. The global predominance of the drum seems to support this belief. Michael Harner summarized his study of global methods of consciousness alteration by stating that throughout most of the world the altered states of consciousness used in shamanism are attained through techniques involving a monotonous percussion sound, most typically done with a drum, but also with sticks, rattles, and other instruments.

Why is the drum such a powerful tool for entering into a shamanic state of consciousness? One possibility is that the drum acts as a focusing device for the shaman. This approach could be compared to various meditation techniques in other traditions where one strives to focus the mind on a specific point. Single-pointed concentration on one object of focus, such as the breath, serves to quiet distracting trains of thought that keep the mind anchored in linear consciousness. The elimination of distracting thoughts is the first stepping stone toward allowing the consciousness to open up to higher states of awareness.

In the shamanic traditions, the drum is often referred to as a type of vehicle that the shaman rides on into the other realms. Phrases such as the shaman "rides his drum like a horse" are found throughout the accounts of shamanic trance journeying experience. The single-pointed focus on the pure sound of the drum is the meditation aid vehicle that transports the shaman's spirit into non-ordinary realities.

Above and beyond its uses as a musical instrument, the drum is considered sacred to the shaman. The instrument is often empowered through ritualistic practices that charge it with powerful energetic intent. Such a drum becomes a potent tool for healing, and, like all tools of power, must be earned. Most sacred drums are given to a drumming adept by their drumming master. The drum is an energy form— a living being working with the shaman to increase his or her power and effectiveness. Such a drum can invoke spirits, chase away diseases, and do magical things. This is a huge topic that could be explored in much more depth. Those of you who would like to delve further into this realm may enjoy following up with Mickey Hart's *Drumming at the Edge of Magic*.

The Science Behind Sound and Altered States

On a physiological level, a more scientific explanation is that drumming stimulates the auditory tracts that pass directly into the reticular activating system (RAS) of the brain. The core function of the RAS is to regulate the general level of electrical activity in the brain. Through a phenomenon known as auditory driving, the sound of drumming creates strong, repetitive neuronal firing in the auditory pathways. Prolonged listening to such sounds serves to overcharge the RAS in a unique way that can greatly reduce, or entirely block out, other sensory stimuli.

This narrowing of the focus of consciousness combined with the high electrical activation of the brain is one physiological explanation for the drum's power to free the shaman's mind to travel to other realms. In a nutshell, the strong repetitive charge of the drumbeat both overloads the more mundane circuits of the brain while simultaneously creating an opening to higher levels of consciousness.

Brain Wave Entrainment

From a broader perspective, this phenomenon of auditory driving is an example of a special type of entrainment. The principles of entrainment can be observed in all varieties of energetic interactions and relationships, but the example here is a type of rhythmic entrainment. The stronger, more persistent, or more coherent source of rhythm or vibration typically influences the other in a way that causes the second system to shift into a state of synchronized pulsation.

On a basic physiological level, breathing and heart rate have been shown to be strongly affected by external sounds, which can have corresponding effects on brain states. The physical sound of the drum is transduced into rhythmic electrical pulses that serve to activate the entire brain in step with the external rhythm. The ability of rhythmic sound to affect human brain wave activity is the essence of auditory driving and is the cause of the resulting altered states of consciousness.

The brain can be entrained to any external rhythm for many different effects. For example, the sound of the heartbeat is very frequently mimicked in shamanic drumming. Heart sounds, particularly of a slow heartbeat, have been proven to be effective in creating responses from listeners similar to anesthesia. The reduced awareness of body sensations and feeling may well serve to free the mind to journey outward. Certain types of yoga and meditation also share this goal. It is first necessary to remove the distraction of body sensations before the consciousness can fully focus on meditative practices. Through the removal of physical distractions, drumming may serve as a powerful ally to assist the shaman in journeying out of the body.

Many shamanic cultures native to both South and North America used very simple beats that are usually around 60 beats per minute or an octave of that (120 beats). However, other traditions use different rhythms. In particular, certain African traditions incorporate very complex, yet very effective rhythms, though they are still based upon the heartbeat. Drums are often the solo instruments in many magical and healing ceremonies in African-based cultures. Powerful examples of percussion-based trance music can be found in the Gnawa and Jajouka traditions of Morocco, both of which support special castes of master musicians with a profound understanding of the magical effects of sound and rhythm. Similar rhythms have developed in or traveled to various parts of the world, such as the heavily African-influenced style of shamanic drumming found in the Vodou tradition of Haiti.

Brain Wave Rhythms

A major aspect of the drum's ability to alter consciousness stems from the fact that our brain waves also pulsate and oscillate at particular frequencies that can be measured, just like sound waves, in cycles per second (or hertz). Therefore the rhythms of sound and states of consciousness are very closely related. There are four basic delineations of different brain wave states based upon the cycles per second of the brain. Brain wave rhythms can be generally corresponded to the following states of awareness and consciousness:

Beta—from 14 to 20 Hz—are found in our normal waking state of consciousness. Beta waves are present when our focus of attention is on activities of the external world.

Alpha—from 8 to 13 Hz—occur when we daydream and are often associated with a state of light meditation. Alpha waves become stronger and more regular when our eyes are closed. Entering alpha begins to allow access to the subconscious realms.

Theta—from 4 to 7 Hz—are found in states of high creativity and have been equated to states of consciousness found in much shamanic work, for this brain wave bandwidth is the range where psychic experiences are most likely to begin to occur. Theta waves are also associated with states of deep meditation and sleep.

Delta—from 0.5 to 3 Hz—typically occur in states of deep sleep or unconsciousness. However, more recent brain wave research indicates that conscious individuals can still actively function in a delta state. This skill is typically only acquired with extensive meditation experience and training of the consciousness.

Laboratory research has verified that drumming produces changes in the central nervous system. Analysis of certain shamanic drumming has revealed that the beats per minute of the rhythms often translate to a range of .8 to 5 cycles per second, which spans between the delta and theta brain wave bandwidths. The rhythmic stimulation affects the electrical activity in various sensory and motor areas of the brain. Many of these centers are not ordinarily connected, but the drum stimulates more holistic connections. This appears to be due in part to the fact that the single beat of a drum contains many sound frequencies, and accordingly it simultaneously transmits impulses along a variety of nerve pathways in the brain. Furthermore, drumbeats are mainly of low frequency. Since the low-frequency receptors of the ear are more resistant to damage than the delicate high-frequency receptors and can withstand higher amplitudes of sound, more energy can be transmitted to the brain via a drumbeat than from a sound stimulus of higher frequency before pain is felt.

The sound of a shamanic drum is one of the fastest ways of inducing altered states of consciousness. One immediately lets go of the everyday thoughts that so constantly keep us from stilling the mind. Perhaps because it is so primal, we respond quickly. The sound of the drum may go straight to that part of our primitive brain that works with pure emotions rather than mentally construed thought. There is no doubt that the entrainment phenomenon affects the heartbeat and other autonomic nervous system functions. However, this factor may be only part of the explanation for the powerful effect of the drum. The musical magic of the drum may find its power in some other answer—perhaps through opening an energetic or psychic gateway to unseen worlds or spirit allies with which the shaman works.

Tools for Shamanic Journeying

Now that we have introduced some fundamental concepts relating to the power of sound to shift levels of awareness, you may wish to make them your own with more direct experience. If you would like to take additional steps into exploring traditional shamanic practice, we once again recommend the work of Michael Harner. In *The Way of the Shaman*, Harner provides instructions and guidelines for the traditional shamanic journeying process and additional guidance to experience the power of sound to shift levels of awareness. While it may be best to venture into the realm of shamanic journeying with a live drummer, that option may be inconvenient for most people. Harner has provided an invaluable service with his recorded shamanic drum offerings that make the power of the drum as a vehicle for sonic journeying available whenever you wish on his shamanic drumming CD called *Shamanic Journey: Solo and Double Drumming.*

Exercise: Shamanic Self-Entrainment

While it would be ideal to experience shamanic drumming entrainment with a live drummer or the substitute of a recording, if you do not have easy access to those options at the moment, here's a quick exercise that will allow you to experience a similar sort of effect now. This exercise will guide you through a process of self-entrainment. For just as external rhythms can shift your heart rate, respiration, and brain waves, your own self-created tones can have a similar effect. This approach can simulate the shamanic drumming experience without requiring an external sound source.

First, find a quiet space in which to make sounds. For this experience, you will simply allow yourself to mimic percussive sounds with your voice. Possible tones could be a *kuh* sound (as in the word "cup") or perhaps a quick *boom* sound simulating the tone of a low-pitched hand drum. For this first experience, we will use the *kuh* sound.

To get started, take a breath and exhale with a short *kuh*. The sound doesn't have to be loud; it can be made at a relaxed low volume. Begin by making the sound once per second until you feel a sense of rhythm begin to lock in. Continue making the sound at this even pace for two to three minutes. Now begin to speed up the rhythm of your sound until it becomes like a fast-paced drumbeat. Continue this for about a minute. Note the difference. You are now in a state of self-entrainment. You have sped up your nervous system.

Next slow down the repetitions, making the percussive sound every two to three seconds. As you do this you will feel your nervous system slow down. Continue for one full minute.

To begin to gauge the effect of this practice on your body rhythms, locate your radial pulse. To find this point, turn your wrist so your palm is facing up. You can feel your radial pulse near where the wrist meets the hand on the side of the thumb. Find the pulse with the index and middle fingers of the other hand.

Once you have found your pulse, you can feel your heartbeat. Try making the *kuh* sounds again, but this time begin by synchronizing your sound with the beat of your heart. As you do this, you are entraining your sound with your heart's present rhythm. Now speed up your sounds so that they are twice as fast as your pulse. See if your heart rate increases. It won't fully speed up to match the pace of your sounds, but it will go faster. Once you have experienced your heart going faster, again slow down the repetitions of your sound so that each *kuh* lasts a full second. Continue this until you notice your heart rate slow noticeably.

After you have had this initial experience, try the exercise again at another time using the *boom* sound. Take note of any differences in the results. For us, the *kuh* sound usually feels energizing, while the *boom* sound feels more relaxing and grounding. Feel free to experiment with other percussive vocal sounds of your choice, and see if you can find others that are even more effective for you.

This exercise shows us the powerful instant feedback system between self-created sound and the body in real time. By entraining ourselves to faster rhythms, we can build internal energy. By slowing ourselves with self-entrainment, we can have a self-soothing effect. These self-created sounds can shift the tempo of your heart rate and respiration. As these body rhythms shift, the brain wave rhythms follow suit, which can result in the first steps toward an altered state of consciousness.

Modern Examples of Consciousness Shifting with Sound

In the preceding sections, we have touched on a few examples of the profound uses of sound in traditional shamanism. This is a vast topic that could be expanded into a much longer work. But now we will move on to introduce an immediate topic—how you can benefit from applying sound and music to your own life utilizing techniques adapted from the ancient wellspring of shamanic practice.

In the realm of traditional shamanism, much of the shaman's work is done in the spirit realms. While we do allow for the reality of nonphysical, spiritual realms and beings, in order to first open the gateway, it may serve to shift the metaphor to the realm of energy. It is possible to view many of the phenomena that have been described throughout human history as "spiritual" in terms of the emerging vocabulary of energy medicine. Many systems of subtle energy work are also very ancient, and it may be of value to strive toward a marriage of energy work practices with the traditional shamanic worldview.

Following this line of thought, the realm in which the modern practitioner begins to work is not so much the spirit realm as the energy field. Energy fields are omnipresent. There are fields of both energy and of consciousness. They surround the body as both electromagnetic fields and more subtle layers of energetic structure. Energetic fields determine the nature and "vibe" of different locations and spaces ranging from one's immediate surroundings to expanding out to a planetary level and beyond.

As we noted in our introduction, sound work can be thought of as a form of energy work. Sound is simply the "densest" bandwidth of subtle energy. Yet the effects and benefits of sound work spiral upward into higher octaves of energy and vibration, perhaps also into the spiritual realm of traditional shamanism. For now we will focus on the role of a sound healer/shamanic practitioner as one who manipulates consciousness and works with energy through sound work techniques. Where does one begin in this realm?

As we have noted, the fundamental skill of the shaman in all traditions is the ability to enter into an altered state of consciousness. We have already discussed how sound can be one of the most profound tools for inducing an altered state. In recent years, various researchers and artists have developed methods for creating recordings capable of inducing specific brain wave states and related states of consciousness. Listening to such specifically crafted recordings could be viewed as a modern means of achieving results that are closely related to the effect produced by shamanic drumming.

Binaural Beat Entrainment

A major pioneer who developed one of the more popular of these modern psychoactive sonic approaches was Robert Monroe. Monroe began his career as a business executive in the field of broadcasting. However, his conservative lifestyle was unexpectedly upset when he began having spontaneous out-of-body experiences in the mid-1960s. These events triggered a fascination with paranormal phenomena and the exploration of consciousness.

Monroe noted that his out-of-body travels seemed to be accompanied by the internal hearing of various ethereal sounds. He began to wonder what role these tones played in actually inducing the experiences. This question inspired him to begin private research into the ability of different frequencies to induce altered states of consciousness. He felt that sound could somehow play a role in helping others achieve similar states of consciousness such as he had experienced, and with the help of a research team, he set out to discover if he could control or drive the brain with sound waves.

Through trial and error, and probably a lot of intuition, Monroe discovered that he could produce a driving or entrainment of brain waves through use of specific sonic techniques. Monroe found that much like a glass that could be resonated by a pure tone, the brain resonated when bombarded with pulsing sound waves. Monroe called this a frequency following response (FFR), and he patented this effect in 1975.

The frequencies that Monroe used to entrain the brain were in the same spectrum as the brain waves themselves—from .5 Hz to about 20 Hz—which are tones below the range of human hearing. However, through the use of a psychoacoustic phenomenon called beat frequencies, Monroe found that it was possible to trigger the brain wave entraining effects of these very low frequencies using much higher audible sound frequencies.

The concept behind the phenomenon is simple: if you use two independent sound sources, say, for example, a tuning fork of 100 Hz, and another tuning fork of 108 Hz, the difference between the two tones will produce a beat frequency (or difference tone) of 8 Hz. However, since it's below the range of human hearing, this new frequency will not be heard as a distinct tone, but it can be perceived as a pulsing *wah-wah-wah* type sound or beat. If the original sounds come from external sources, such as two separate loudspeakers, these beats can be heard and felt via normal open-air listening. This basic manifestation of the phenomenon is called a monaural beat frequency.

Monroe took the basic beat frequency effect even further. If the two different frequencies are applied separately to each ear via headphones, a binaural beat frequency is created. This beat frequency is not an actual sound but a phenomenon created within the brain itself based on the difference between the two actual sounds heard by each ear. The remarkable result is that the brain wave rhythms will entrain to the difference tone between the two frequencies. Thus, a tone of 100 Hz in one ear and a tone of 108 Hz in the other will cause the brain wave rhythms to pulse at the 8 Hz difference, resulting in an alpha brain wave pattern. Similarly, frequencies of 100 Hz and 104 Hz introduced separately via headphones will create a 4 Hz brain wave entrainment in the theta wave bandwidth. In a nutshell, the brain can be entrained to any difference tone created by two separate stereo frequencies introduced via headphones.

Benefits of Brain Wave Entrainment

Entraining the brain to specific wavelengths can have many benefits, but in relation to our consideration of shamanism, it is conceivable that the phenomenon can help facilitate communion with sources of intelligence and information that would be difficult to access in normal states of consciousness. The basic concept is that the mind could be thought of as a type of radio receiver. If one can shift the rhythm of brain wave patterns to match specific outside frequencies, then one can conceptually open the consciousness to interact with these frequencies via a type of psychic sympathetic resonance.

One popular example is the Schumann Resonance effect. The sound of Earth, or more accurately the frequency of Earth's ionosphere (which is the electromagnetic field around Earth), is known as the Schumann Resonance. Although the Schumann Resonance modulates over a wide range of frequencies, it has been measured to average around 7.8 cycles per second. This frequency falls within the alpha wave spectrum of the human brain. It has been speculated that when our brain waves sync up with this frequency, it is possible to entrain with the energies of Earth.

In his book *Stalking the Wild Pendulum*, Itzhak Bentov was one of the first to propose that when a person begins to enter this 7.8 cycle per second brain wave state during meditation, it would conceivably be possible to lock in resonance with Earth's frequency. He believed that this resonant connection could serve to expand consciousness to greater fields of perception and information. Indeed, research has shown that psychics often generate brain waves in the 7–8 Hz range while attempting to produce certain paranormal phenomenon.

It has also been suggested by the pioneering researcher into the subtle electromagnetic fields of the body, Dr. Robert O. Becker, that perhaps this Earth frequency is a "cosmic carrier wave of information" and could be the "drummer" to which these psychics, healers, dowsers, etc. were entrained. He found that this brain wave bandwidth of 7.8 Hz makes subjects more open to a variety of information sources, including those associated with paranormal phenomenon.[12] Therefore, working within this brain wave bandwidth would be of great value to those involved with subtle energetic healing arts, for this state could serve to dramatically increase awareness and sensitivity to subtle flows of energy. The effect may be further enhanced by brain wave rhythms in the theta and delta bandwidths, but the ability to operate consciously in these states may require slightly more advanced levels of training. In any case, a simple way to begin to explore this realm is via high-quality brain wave entrainment recordings.

The Future May Be Found in the Past?

Brain wave entrainment has only gained popular awareness since the 1970s. Yet the phenomenon of sonic entrainment

---

12. Robert O. Becker and Gary Selden, *The Body Electric: Electromagnetism and the Foundation of Life* (New York: Morrow, 1985).

has been used by medicine people and shamans from different cultures since prehistoric times. If we analyze the auditory aids utilized by shamans to induce altered states of consciousness, they reveal a sophistication of techniques that modern science in the form of technologies such as Hemi-Sync have only recently begun to realize.

The ability to create altered states of consciousness through drumming, chanting, and music is probably as old as music itself. Through driving the brain with various specific sounds, the shaman is able to induce much the same effect as much of the scientific technology discussed above. But in addition to the drum, a number of other sound-generating tools utilized in ancient cultures provide even more thought-provoking evidence of a profound awareness of the consciousness altering power of brain wave entrainment sound. Therefore, these modern discoveries related to brain wave entrainment may simply be a reawakening of ancient knowledge of how sound can be used to shift states of consciousness.

One easily accessible example of a sound tool that demonstrates this belief is Tibetan bells, or tingshas. These bells have been utilized in Buddhist meditation practice for many centuries. An examination reveals that the two bells, which are rung together, are slightly out of tune with each other. Depending upon the bells, the difference tones between them create low frequencies somewhere between 4 and 8 cycles per second. This falls exactly within the range of the brain waves created during meditation and helps shift the brain to these frequencies. It is little wonder that tingshas are experiencing a worldwide increase in popularity as tools for increased relaxation and reduction of stress.

Tingshas are readily available in many Tibetan gift shops and various mind/body/spirit type stores. However, note that the craftsmanship of the sets is highly irregular. To judge them, ting them gently together and listen for the beat frequency pulse that they produce. Cheap bells will often have an unsettling speedy pulse. But higher quality sets produce a relaxing slow beat. Every set will sound different, but your own taste will ultimately be the judge. Try a number of different choices to find a set that feels best to you.

Peruvian whistling vessels offer another fascinating demonstration of ancient sonic knowledge. These vessels are pipelike instruments originally found buried with mummies in Peru. Conventional anthropologists originally believed that they were just ornate drinking vessels. Thanks to later research initiated by the pioneering discoveries of Daniel Statnekov in the 1970s, the vessels were revealed to be profound psychoacoustic instruments. The vessels are traditionally blown in carefully tuned sets of seven. Each individual vessel produces a high-pitched whistling tone that does not sound very noteworthy in isolation. Yet when blown together, the ensemble produces an entrancing symphony of interweaving beat frequencies. The sound produced by a full set of Peruvian whistling vessels has been likened to a sort of sonic psychotropic, for they often trigger intense altered states and vivid visionary experiences in listeners.

Although their exact usage in ancient times is still a mystery, it seems highly likely that these vessels were sacred tools, probably used under the guidance of a shaman or a priest and utilized only at specific times and for ritual purposes. Listening to these whistling vessels makes one truly appreciate the possibility of profound knowledge of sound among ancient cultures.

The Peruvian whistling vessels and the Tibetan bells are two examples of shamanic tools that employ the concept of sonic entrainment for the brain. Numerous other ancient cultures clearly knew of these principles for using specialized beat frequencies to alter consciousness and applied them in their instruments, drumming, and chanting. Today, healers and therapists working with sound and music have the potential of following in the paths of the ancient shamanic traditions, combining magic and mysticism with modern science and technology. It truly is an exciting era of new possibilities! The current accessibility of both ancient knowledge and cutting-edge brain science offers many creative options to modern sonic shamanic practitioners.

What Is an Altered State?

We have so far discussed listening to specially created psychoacoustic recordings and instruments to induce altered states of consciousness. Exploring these approaches is highly recommended, but note that outside aids are not completely mandatory. As we can recall from the exercises and examples from the previous chapter, it is possible to create an altered state through focused listening at any time. An altered state does not necessary have to be a dramatic mystical excursion. In fact, the precise definition of such a state is somewhat vague. It can be as simple as shifting into a different state than the one previously occupied a moment before. In reality, we all shift among states of consciousness all day long! For example, when engaged in focused work we are in a certain state (typically a beta state), but if you take a few moments off to shift attention elsewhere, say to gaze out the window for a few minutes, you may find yourself shifting into more of an alpha brain wave pattern. Which was a different state than the one previously occupied.

In reality, there may be no such thing as a "normal" state of consciousness. We all shift through such a wide array of emotions and mental states throughout any given day, there's no firm basis to declare any one of them to be "normal." The key is to learn to become more observant of subtle shifts in one's state of consciousness. As one becomes more aware of such changes, one can become more skillful at making such shifts at will. This awareness also provides the foundation for learning to deepen and enhance one's altered states, and perhaps it is also the gateway toward the more profound journeys in consciousness experienced by the shamanic practitioner. In the essay "The Trance of Healing" from his book *Shamans, Healers, and Medicine Men*, Holger Kalweit echoes this belief saying:

> *Human existence is open in all directions for experiences of consciousnesses of all kinds. We continually swing back and forth on a consciousness continuum between subwakeful and hyperconscious states. Indeed, we live in a mercurial universe of consciousness. This leads to a conception of the psyche as a journey through various zones of consciousness. I believe it is one of our tasks to learn to distinguish these states clearly from one*

*another in such a way that we can become masters of our
own "creations."* 13

Here we have the essential skill—the ability to modulate
your consciousness in order to achieve various desired results.
Sound can be a powerful ally toward this goal. Since many
of us are primarily visual in nature, simply shifting greater
awareness to the world of sound is often enough to begin
to induce a trance state. Many people spend the majority of
their day in "left brain" linear activities such as reading, writing, or mathematical tasks. The shift into the different sensory
modality of enhanced auditory awareness involves entering
into an altered state. Once that shift is made, one can progress
through different levels of awareness that can deepen your
experience of the sonic environment that surrounds us at
all times and enhance your ability to interact with it in more
consciously chosen beneficial ways.

You may wish to revisit the chapter 3 listening exercises
with the new perspectives offered in this chapter. These seemingly simple exercises can yield many new plateaus of insight,
and you may find that they can serve as even more powerful
triggers for opening to the type of journeying enjoyed by the
shamanic practitioner. In any case, we hope we have inspired a
few new ideas regarding how you can begin to shift your own
energy states and consciousness through the power of sound.
And in this spirit we will now move on to consider the active
practice of vocal toning, which is one of the most powerful
tools we have available to modulate and cultivate our own
energy states.

---

13. Holger Kalweit, *Shamans, Healers, and Medicine Men* (Boston:
    Shambhala, 1992), 81.

Recommended Reading

Brain States by Tom Kenyon

Drumming at the Edge of Magic: A Journey into the Spirit of Percussion by Mickey Hart and Jay Stevens

Imagery in Healing: Shamanism and Modern Medicine by Jeanne Achterberg

Stalking the Wild Pendulum: On the Mechanics of Consciousness by Itzhak Bentov

The Way of the Shaman by Michael Harner

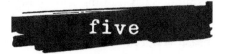

five

Vocal Toning Part One

The Energetics of Breath

> *A bird does not sing because it has an answer,*
> *it sings because it has a song.*
> —ANCIENT CHINESE PROVERB

Sound healing is a vast field. Where should one begin in order to grasp its many niches and nuances? To recap, sound is an energy form that we experience most palpably on the physical plane—audible energy. Yet it's quickly capable of forming a bridge between the realms of energetic intention and physical manifestation. Sound is a creative force, and ultimately an intelligent force.

As we noted at the end of chapter 2, sound can be discussed and analyzed in terms of frequency analysis. But we feel that in order to begin to understand it on the most expansive levels, it's useful to first step back to a more holistic perspective that honors the full multidimensional aspects of sound. The more analytical perspectives can then be brought back into play more constructively after a fuller grounding in the totality of sound. Such training and knowledge should always be in service to the perspective that the highest role of the sound healer is not merely to project or perform consciously contrived frequencies but to be an open channel, or instrument, for the therapeutic and transformative powers of sound.

This intention is summed up very well by St. Francis in his prayer "Oh Lord, make me an instrument." Here the thought form is that one is not the primary source of the healing energy but the conduit through which it flows. Another example of this perspective can be found in the popular energy work modality of Reiki. Reiki is a form of energy medicine originally from Japan that has gained notoriety and popularity in the West. A large part of Reiki training consists of various attunements that permit one to channel the Reiki current. The practitioner is not the primary generator of the Reiki energy but aspires to become a pure conduit for it to flow through, i.e., an instrument.

In the realm of sound, one also has the powerful ability to physically generate the fundamental energy. This advantage is significant because, in and of itself, physical plane sound has the ability to shape and rearrange molecules and cells and create various physical and energetic structures. This phenomenon has been well demonstrated in the science of cymatics.

In a nutshell, the cymatics work documents the profoundly thought-provoking fact that sound creates form! The term was coined by Dr. Hans Jenny, a visionary Swiss medical doctor who in his spare time spent many hours observing and investigating the effects of sound upon matter. Many consider this work to be the most important documentation of the ability of sound to shape substance.

His seminal work entitled *Cymatics* (derived from the Greek word *kyma*, which means "wave") shows the effects of sound frequencies upon many different types of material, including water, pastes, liquids, and plastics. Dr. Jenny placed these substances on a steel plate, vibrated the plate with a crystal oscillator, which produced an exact frequency, and then photographed the effects. The many different shapes that he photographed included pictures of a liquid plastic material that morphed into very lifelike, organic-looking structures. Lycopodium dust (a material like talcum powder) took on shapes resembling the cells of the body, and water took on many extraordinary geometric forms depending upon the frequency projected into it. The cymatics images produced by Dr. Jenny and his followers truly bring the insights from this field of study to life.[14]

In spite of the easily observable effects of basic physical sound, the real magic begins to occur when sound is combined with focused consciousness or intention. Then the physical waveforms of sound become potently charged with the intent of the practitioner, which opens the gateway to weaving in the powerful synergy of techniques and insights gleaned from other energy medicine modalities. Thus, it is not merely the sound (or the frequency) that one generates, but the energy of the intentionality that one transmits on it. This is a multilayered and nuanced concept that we will develop more in chapter 9.

---

14. To see images, visit www.cymatics.org.

We feel that the best starting point to begin to understand the complexity of sound is via immersion in the accessible physical plane vibration of sound. It's an experiential, not informational, learning approach that invites sound itself to become your primary teacher and the direct sound current to become the primary source of initiation.

In order to accomplish this goal, the approach we will focus on is the practice of vocal toning. Toning has many definitions, but we will simply think of it as the practice of making sustained sounds with the voice for therapeutic and meditative purposes.

Toning can most expansively be thought of as the practice of generating and shaping pure energy in the form of sound via the voice. The human voice offers great advantages over the multitude of external instruments created for healing and transformational effects. The voice does not require batteries, electricity, or external sound sources. It's the one tool that is most natural, easiest to learn to use, and free to access! As a form of energy work, vocal toning is unique; the effects and benefits of toning are intimately unique to each individual utilizing powerful but gentle self-created sounds do not take you beyond a place you are ready to assimilate.

Exercise: Yawn/Sigh

Before we begin to explore vocal toning more systematically, let's begin with a quick experience. The gateway to toning work can be opened by the simple sounds that we make naturally. The yawn/sigh exercise is a simple technique to introduce what it's like to shift your energy state with sound.

To begin, sit comfortably with your spine erect. Take a moment to assess your current state. Without analyzing too much, just tune in and take a quick snapshot of how you feel at the moment. Next, take a deep breath, hold it for a few seconds, and then release it with a sigh. Now repeat. Take another full, deep breath and release it with a drawn-out sigh. Let your sigh last longer than before, and as you exhale feel that you are releasing all tension with your sound. Now do it a third time. This time, take an even deeper breath and release it with an even louder and longer, more drawn-out sigh.

After these three rounds, take note of how you feel now. Do you feel any energy shift, no matter how slight? Perhaps you feel more relaxed, centered, or grounded in your body?

To enhance the effect of this technique, try the following variation. When you breathe in, make your inhale an exaggerated deep yawn. As you yawn, open your jaw as wide as possible. Hold your jaw open as you hold your breath for a few seconds. When you release with the sigh, let the tone of your sigh sweep from a high to a low pitch. Repeat two more times, letting your sigh last slightly longer with each repetition.

How do you feel now? Just simply allowing yourself to make natural sounds is the most basic essence of vocal toning. Many people find this simple exercise to be an effective technique to help release tension and relax. It can be done anywhere, anytime, throughout the day to give yourself a quick energy reset. And it can also serve as a tension releasing warm-up for some of the exercises we will offer later in this chapter.

Basic Vocal Toning Concepts

Engaging in the personal practice of vocal toning can be a powerful journey of self-discovery. Over the gates of Delphi, where the Grecian Oracle dwelt, it read: "Know Thyself." There is no better way of gaining safe access into greater understanding of your own being than through self-created sounds. In the upcoming pages, you will be guided through an experiential journey through your own resonances, both physically and energetically. In addition to the invaluable self-awareness that will result from this process, this exploration will trigger insights about how sound may be used on others. The most profound insights about how sound may be applied therapeutically come from first experiencing the vibrations in the personal laboratory of your own body and energy field.

Through learning to use our voice as an instrument for healing and self-transformation, we can learn to resonate our physical body and energy centers such as our chakras with our own sounds. It's true that there are also a number of different electronic instruments and recordings that claim to be able to accomplish these effects. Yet, in order to assess the validity of these methods, we would ask you to consider one fundamental question: do all beings vibrate at the same frequency?

In order to speculate on this question, it is necessary to recall the basic premise of sound healing—which is that everything in the universe is in a state of vibration, from the page you are reading to the chair you may be sitting on. Everything that is in a state of motion is vibrating, and therefore is creating a sound, at least on the subtle energy level. This includes, of course, your body. Every organ, bone, and tissue is vibrating at particular frequencies. When we are in a state of health, the body is vibrating at an overall composite frequency of all these other different frequencies, like a harmonious chord of resonance. When we are in a state of imbalance, some part of our body is vibrating outside its natural frequency, and we call this "disease." One of the first principles of sound healing is that it may be possible to cause that which is vibrating out of its natural resonance to return to its normal frequency by working with sound, thus restoring overall harmony to the whole being.

As noted, there are a number of different instruments, machines, devices, and CDs that work off this principle, all claiming to have the correct resonant frequency for what ails you, whether it be a part of the physical body or an energy center such as a particular chakra. It becomes interesting to note that these frequencies, depending upon their source, can often vary widely. In spite of the seeming contradictions, different frequency sets often seem to have successful results within their given practitioners' frameworks. This may be due to the possibility that vibrational rates for various organs and structures may truly vary from person to person. It may also be that the personal energy of the healer may be more responsible for the healing effect than the surface level protocol of the treatment. Nevertheless, we can observe a number of different systems that employ specific sound frequencies for healing that do not match. That is the first thought to consider.

Issue number two brings us back to the question—do all beings vibrate at the same frequency? At present, no one really knows. It is certainly interesting to consider that perhaps we do not all vibrate at the same frequencies. Perhaps we are all unique vibratory beings! There may well be generic frequencies that would operate within a general range that would work with organs such as the liver or the heart, but the exact frequencies may really vary from person to person. A therapeutic instrument that is limited to the specific frequencies correlated into its design may be effective on a general level, but it will certainly never be capable of the endless variety and specificity that the human voice is capable of evoking.

Through learning to use our voices, it is possible that we can get very specific with the finely tuned sounds that are most appropriate for our own unique resonances. We can also make spontaneous adjustments for ongoing shifts in our personal vibrational rate. This empowered flexibility is extremely important and may need a word of explanation.

For example, if we are locked in the belief system that energy structures such as our chakras all vibrate to particular fixed frequencies, there is not much room for shift, change, and evolution. The goal for the exercises in this book is to provide the opportunity for you to explore your own resonances through the power of your own voice. The sounds that you create will be the primary teachers.

For the most part, exercises will mainly be presented without much explanation. Your own direct experience with the sound current will be your primary source of initiation and instruction. Doing the exercises without any preconditioning relating to the effects will open you up to a much wider range of possible experiences. This exploration is not structured with prescriptive teaching such as "make sound X and expect Y to happen." The goal is to simply make the sounds. You are being empowered to simply create the sounds, and tune in mindfully to your own responses and resonances. Your reactions will be unique for you as an individual, but they will also provide insights into the wide variety of effects and experiences that vocal toning can provide.

The experiences that result from the same sets of exercises will vary greatly from individual to individual. Sound is a multidimensional energy form. Sounding can affect us on the physical, energetic, emotional, and spiritual levels. Be open to noticing experiences on all of these planes, but, above all, do not judge yourself by some preconceived standard of expectation as to what may result. Simply note what does happen. For example, some people may focus on physical or energetic sensations, whereas others may experience powerful emotional events from the same exercise. Whatever happens is what is right and proper for you at that particular time. You may be surprised to find that if you do any given sonic exercise at a different time and space, you may have different reactions or another layer of experience.

May the following pages serve as an initiation into the wonders of the sound current that can be invoked and evoked through the power of your own voice. We look forward to accompanying you on this exciting sonic journey!

The Foundation of Vocal Toning: Breath Awareness

Before we begin the active toning work exercises, the first topic to consider is the awareness of the power of breath. A grounding in conscious breathwork provides an essential foundation for effective toning. Information about breathwork and proper breathing approaches is available from a number of sources. Even if the concepts are not new to you, we encourage you to review these practices from a fresh perspective as a precursor to the toning work. For breath is not only the energy source that will fuel the power of your toning, it is also a potent category of toning in and of itself. The contemplation and practice of breathwork as a type of subtle energy toning could well yield new insights.

Breath is simply the foundation of all life! While one could exist for a number of days without food and perhaps several days without water, one could not go without taking a breath for more than a few minutes, at best. In addition to being the main nourishment that sustains physical life, breath is the root force for all of the subtle energy systems.

The terms for the body's subtle energy currents vary from tradition to tradition. It is called *chi* in Chinese terminology, *ki* in Japanese, *ruach* in Hebrew, and *prana* in the Ayurvedic traditions. All of these terms are basically synonymous, or have direct linguistic roots, to the words for breath. Even our English word *spirit* derives from the Greek term "spiritus," which also means breath. When people use the word *spiritual*, they are often attempting to describe an experience or a condition that is above and beyond ordinary physical experience or a state of consciousness or awareness that is expanded beyond our average/common daily state. The breath could quite rightly be viewed as the vehicle that forms the bridge between the mundane and the spiritual.

The skills of proper breathing have many benefits, for basic modulation of your breath can serve to shift your physiology, heart rate, brain waves, and ultimately, your state of consciousness. The yoga of breath, or pranayama, is a vast and intricate set of practices that would warrant a separate program in their own right. But for our purposes here, we will introduce some fundamental approaches that will serve to enhance your vocal toning ability, which will continue to develop as you advance through the exercises in the following pages.

As we continue to expand on the concepts of vocal toning, it is important to note that a distinction must be made between toning and performance singing. Our program is not to be viewed as a singing course, yet these two forms of vocalization share a common foundation—the breath.

Throughout these pages, we will stress a number of times that all sounds should be made in whatever range you are currently comfortable with. One should never force or strain to hit any sound. As you proceed, you may find that this range will expand. One way to accomplish this goal is through greater attention to the breath.

Exercise: Abdominal Breathing

As with performance singing, the simple, practical goal pertaining to breath in the realm of toning is to be able to breathe in such a way that will enable you to sustain your tone for as long as is desired. As stated above, one should never strain or force, but being able to sustain your tone for longer durations will often enhance your experience with the sounding.

The first step to consider is your intake of breath. Before we continue, stop and take a breath as you are naturally inclined to do. Which parts of your body do you feel expanding as you take air in? Now exhale fully. Pause for a count of three before taking another breath. This step may make you more mindful of the subtle sensations involved with breathing in.

Now place one hand gently on your lower rib cage and the other on your navel. Repeat the above process—exhale fully, count to three, and then inhale again. Did you feel either of the areas under your hands expanding as you breathed in? Perhaps you felt the lower ribs expand as you took your breath. Perhaps you felt your abdomen expand, as well. If so, very good! But if you did not feel your stomach expand, or if your stomach sucked in while inhaling, this is the first area we would like to improve on.

A full, complete breath involves attention to the practice of abdominal breathing. As you breathe in, your abdomen should expand with air. Place your hand on your navel again and take another breath. Your abdomen should expand as you take your in breath. One should not force the abdomen out on the inhale, but rather you should allow this area to relax and expand naturally to accommodate the incoming air.

It may be helpful to imagine to slow down the duration of your inhale. Imagine that the incoming air is like a heavy fluid that is being poured in to fill your whole torso. Imagine and feel that the lowest point being filled by this fluid is the region below your navel. As you inhale, feel the area between your hips and lower ribs expand with the in breath while simultaneously allowing your stomach to expand outward.

Note that this technique may feel awkward at first, which is understandable. In Western culture, we have all been conditioned to feel self-conscious about having flat stomachs. This phenomenon often results in the tendency to suck in our stomachs, either unconsciously or very deliberately, in sometimes extreme ways. It's time to let this habit go. You now have permission to let your stomach expand freely. Relax and let it go! No one is watching!

As you continue to practice, abdominal breathing will begin to feel completely natural. You may even feel a sense of "returning home" because it is the most natural and efficient way to breathe and the fashion that supplies the body with the greatest charge of energy.

Exercise: Alternate Breath Awareness Practice

Many people find it helpful to become accustomed to the sensation of abdominal breathing while lying down. You may wish to try this practice in addition to the one described above.

To begin, first lie on your back. Do a gentle partial sit-up (or abdominal crunch) to help increase awareness of your midsection. This motion does not have to be very strenuous, just enough to lift your shoulders off the ground by an inch or two. As you lower your shoulders back to the floor, keep your abdominal muscles tensed and hold for an extra second or two. Then release the tension in your stomach area with a quick, releasing sigh.

Repeat this practice two to three times. That should be all it takes to begin to feel a more relaxed sensation in your abdominal region. When you believe that you've got it, place your hand on your navel and do a gentle measured inhale through your nose. As you do so, imagine that there is a balloon in your stomach that is slowly being filled with the incoming air. If done properly, you should feel your hand begin to rise and continue to do so throughout the in breath. On the exhale, feel with your hand how the belly sinks back down with the release of air.

Inhalation

While the technique of abdominal breathing is crucially important, it is worth noting that if you are only breathing abdominally, it's still an incomplete breath! The issue is not nearly as common as the (more serious) problem of high upper chest breathing that is common amongst people who have not been introduced to mindful breathwork practices, but it's worth noting.

One could analyze the subtleties of breath in many ways. Indeed, whole books have been written on the subject of pranayama (the yoga of breathwork), but for our purposes it is useful to think of the inhale as having three components.

The first part is the abdominal breath, as described above. Filling the belly with air sets you up for the highest volume intake of breath. The second piece is mindfulness to filling the lungs. At around the point where it feels like the stomach area is about half filled to capacity, begin to shift your attention higher and feel your lower ribs begin to expand as the belly continues to rise. Keep inhaling as you allow your attention to shift even higher, all the way up throughout your chest. When your lungs have reached their full capacity, you should feel a pleasant expansion, or stretching outward, of all your ribs. As with beginning abdominal breathing, doing this practice in a mindful way may seem awkward or uncomfortable at first, but it will become smoother and more natural as you proceed.

The third area to tune in to is around the collarbone and the base of the throat. At the end of a truly full inhale, you should feel an expanding sensation under the collarbone, followed by a gentle sense of pressure as the base of your throat fills with air. This last stage will feel a bit like the sensation of yawning, but here it is the last component of a full inhale, rather a separate type of inhale. To isolate the area, you may find it helpful to do a few yawns as a separate practice. Note the pleasant sensation as your throat and upper chest fill with air.

Exercise: The Inhale Breath Practice

Set aside fifteen minutes to practice the types of breathing. Split your time between the upright and lying down positions. As with all exercises, the first goal is to never stress or strain yourself. If you are new to this type of breathwork, take care to stay within your comfortable limits. As you proceed, you will find that these limits will begin to expand.

Breathwork and pranayama are very intricate and detailed fields of practice. Our goal here is to simply increase awareness of breath in order to maximize air intake to support the practice of vocal toning.

As you breathe in, let your attention shift between the three focal points of the inhale described above. As a general rule of thumb, concentrate first on the abdominal pull of breath. When that region feels like it is about half full, shift your awareness up to the ribs and begin to focus on filling that region with air. Note that you will still be simultaneously filling the abdomen while phasing into the lung expansion.

When the lungs feel like they are about 90 percent filled with air, shift your attention to the collarbone and base of the throat region, allowing that section to expand. When that area is full, you should feel that pleasant expansion in the lower throat. The full inhale is complete when all three regions hit their fullest point simultaneously. Take note of what it feels like to be completely filled with air. Gently hold your breath for two or three seconds, and then allow the air to exhale with a gradual relaxing of the diaphragm.

Have fun with this exploration of breath! In a very real way, this is the first step to consciously manipulating your life force energy! View the practice outlined in the paragraph above as a suggested approach only. You may also wish to try concentrating on the inhale sequence in the opposite order as described. You could also try focusing on the three components of the inhale in varying orders or in isolation. In doing so, you will experience many insights into the subtleties of breathing. You can allow your own current of breath to be your teacher. Enjoy!

Exhalation

In the previous section, we focused on the foundation of breathwork—the inhale. But now it's time to consider the obvious third component—the exhale! Both elements are crucial for your vocal toning practice. Being able to fill yourself completely with air provides the energy for your sounding, but being able to control your release of air will allow you to support your tones in an ideal way and make it possible for you to sustain whatever duration of sounding that you wish to achieve.

As we take the first steps into this practice, comparisons may immediately come to mind relating to singing practice, but we find it useful to conceive of vocal toning as a separate category of vocalization. The first two are normal speech and singing. We view vocal toning as a third category of vocalization. Although toning shares many elements in common with the other two types of articulation, we like to think of it as the third voice.

Toning may share many basic technical elements with singing, but it is worth noting again that it is a very different practice. Performance-oriented singing is many things to many people, but it is often largely concerned with artistic and personal expression. It is useful to think of toning as a more impersonal practice. In this realm, you are simply using the voice as a means to generate and manipulate energy in the form of sound created by your own voice. Toning can definitely take on dimensions of personal expression, and it can be used as a powerful means of shifting and working with emotional energy, but these are more specialized practices that can be addressed after gaining experience with the foundations.

For now, at the beginning, it can be very liberating to think of the voice simply as a detached sound source. This perspective can help bypass any inhibiting self-judgments about vocal quality, and/or one's perceived ability about not being able to sing well. But the sneaky thing about engaging in a vocal toning practice is that there are often spillover benefits in terms of improvements to both the speaking and singing voices.

To return to our current theme, the release of breath is the common denominator to consider with all three types of vocalization. As is particularly important with good singing practice, with toning one should only allow the release of air necessary to support your vocal tone. There is a fine balance to be achieved between not releasing enough air for a strong tone, and releasing too much. Working with the following exercises may be helpful in regulating the exhale in order to achieve the quality and duration of tones that you desire.

In certain types of yogic breathing exercises, attention is often paid to breathing in a measured way. Typically, one inhales to a certain counted rhythm and exhales in alignment with the same even count. The lengths can vary, with the exhale usually being longer than the inhale. The pauses between the inhale and exhale can also figure into the practice. According to some sources, an ideal yogic breath consists of inhaling to a count of four, retaining the breath for a count of eight, and exhaling to a count of sixteen.

This ratio may have profound benefits to energize the body and cleanse your system, but we will be concentrating on a slightly more simplified approach. Our concern now is simply to increase your awareness of breath regulation in order to support your toning practice.

Exercise: The Exhale Breath Practice

Begin this exercise with a few minutes worth of full deep breathing as in the previous exercise. When you feel that you are breathing completely in a relaxed way, begin to establish a count. The count should be at a steady, regular rhythm, with multiples of four often being a useful measure. The rhythm should be a medium pace, perhaps one count per second. If you wish to maintain an even pace without having to worry about the timing of your counting, you could try the practice with a metronome. Inexpensive metronomes should be readily available at any music store.

Begin with a relatively quick inhale and exhale. Make them the same duration. Inhale fully to a count of four, and exhale to a count of four. Be sure to release all breath evenly on the exhale. Repeat this sequence several times until it feels comfortable and natural.

Next, make the inhale and exhale longer, in time with the same rhythm. Inhale to a count of eight, and exhale to a count of eight. Tune in to any reactions you may have. Does this longer count feel different than the first approach? How so?

After getting a feel for breathing at an even pace, begin to vary the length of the exhale. Try making the exhale twice as long as the inhale. Begin with inhaling to a count of four and exhaling to a count of eight. After that ratio begins to feel comfortable, try inhaling to a count of eight and exhaling to a count of sixteen.

Continue with these exercises for at least ten or fifteen minutes. The goal will be to continue to increase the length of the exhale. If you can reach the point where you can sustain the length of the exhale to three times the duration of the inhale, you will be doing well. Four times or longer would be excellent.

Please note, once again, that you should never force or strain your breathing! Do not try to heroically sustain the exhale beyond what is currently comfortable. If longer exhale ratios feel difficult, stick with the counts that are easy to sustain. Your ability will improve as you continue to practice. Also note that you could achieve slightly longer exhales by simply doing a slower count, rather than by doubling the ratios as described above.

Have fun with these breath exercises! It would be advisable to continue to work with measured rhythmic breathing practices on a regular basis for at least a week or two. If you accomplish that goal, you may well notice permanent changes in your breathing patterns that will have holistic benefits on your daily energy levels and states. Indeed, there are many practitioners who spend their whole lives on mindfulness of breath practice. There are endless new layers and plateaus to be discovered. Above all, remember that breath is not only the support system for your vocal toning practices, it is the most basic, fundamental sound that we all utter every day throughout our lives, from the first inhale immediately after emerging from the womb to the last breath that merges with the universe at the end of our days.

Recommended Reading

Conscious Breathing: Breathwork for Health, Stress Release, and Personal Mastery by Gay Hendricks

Cymatics: A Study of Wave Phenomena and Vibration by Hans Jenny

Science of Breath: A Practical Guide by Swami Rama

The Yoga of Breath: A Step-by-Step Guide to Pranayama by Richard Rosen and Kim Fraley

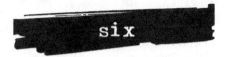

six

Vocal Toning Part Two

The Energetics of Voice

*In speaking, toning or chanting, with knowing and
conviction, we are able to bring oneness to our divided nature.
We are made whole.*

—LAUREL ELIZABETH KEYS

N ow that we have some foundational grounding with
the subtleties of breath, it's time to take our first steps
into the realm of vocal toning. We will begin with the simple
introductory experience of adding some subtle sound to the
inhalations and exhalations. The bridge between breathwork
and active sounding is a fascinating realm to explore. Consider these exercises to be just an introduction.

The breath really is the first and most fundamental of
all tones. Consider how the breathing is always a reflection
of one's emotional and energetic state. How do you breathe
while feeling relaxed and calm? How do you breathe when
excited or agitated or when feeling stressed?

Begin with regulated breathing, as in the previous breath exercise. For this exercise, we will use a simple even ratio of eight counts for the inhale, eight counts for the exhale. Simply breathe in and out for several minutes, focusing your attention on the breath while listening to the sounds you are creating naturally.

When you are ready, begin to put some gentle sound on the breath. These will be gentle aspirated sounds, just quietly accentuating and shaping the natural sounds of your breath.

Begin by adding an *sss* sound as you inhale, followed by and *hhh* sound on the exhale. Allow the first sound to be sort of like a gentle hissing, and the second to be a very breathy *hhhhaaa*, with emphasis on the *hhh* part of the syllable.

Alternate between these sounds for several minutes, and then reverse them. Do the *hhh* sound on the inhale, and the *sss* on the exhale. Tone this new combination for several minutes.

Take note of any differences you may have felt between the two approaches. Did you feel any shift in your experience or energy just from this subtle variation in the inflection of your breath? There is a valuable lesson here that subtle shifts in quiet sounds can still have profound energetic effects. Louder is not always better!

Toning Approach One: Humming

We will now proceed with our journey into vocal toning. You may have already had some powerful experiences and insights just working with the breath, and we encourage you to continue with breathwork exercises on an ongoing basis. But now we are going to begin to engage the voice box. This evolution provides the real initiations into the power of self-created sounds.

At this point, it's worth repeating that vocal toning is not a singing practice! In this style of vocalization, we are going to think of the voice simply as a generator of vibratory energy. You may release any judgments or inhibitions you may have about the aesthetic quality of your vocal sounds. Instead, begin to enjoy the liberating feeling of freedom as you open up and let your own unique voice become a conduit for the energy of sound.

Before we begin sounding, please remember one of the most important aspects of sound work, which is to always honor silence. You may recall profound experiences with the listening exercises from a previous session—these types of experiences are always enhanced after active sound. Please allow the time to experience and enjoy a period of silent meditation after every type of sound-creating exercise, especially after doing internalized vocal toning. It is in these periods of silence, after the physical sound has ceased, that the most profound shifts and changes often occur. Although the audible sound may have ceased, the vibrations you have created will continue to resonate energetically. Many people find this period of silence to be the most profound aspect of any sound work session.

Exercise: Simple Humming

We will begin with one of the most accessible and universal of all sounds, the simple practice of humming. Although seemingly simple, humming may actually be one of the most profound toning practices! Perhaps its greatest importance is that it's really our most inwardly directed sound, and in that aspect has its greatest strength as a sonic resonator of our bodies. Many people believe it is the most powerful sound for creating an "internal massage" of your body—from your internal organs (including your brain) to your muscles and even your nervous system. Most other vocal sounds are primarily outwardly directed. Only the hum—the sound made totally and completely with the mouth closed—is totally inwardly directed. For all its seeming simplicity, there are many veteran sound workers who find the hum to be the most profoundly healing sound of them all.

There is really not much instruction necessary in order to hum. First, simply say the word *hum*. Sustain the *mmm* sound at the end with closed lips and you're doing it! Like many simple-seeming practices, there are endless levels of subtle exploration via the hum.

Find a comfortable place to sit where you can make sounds and not be disturbed. This is important because many times it is necessary to focus our attention on the sounds you are creating in order to feel them. In addition, it is often a good idea to tone with your eyes closed. This seems to enhance our ability to experience the power of our self-created sounds. It's also good to keep your back as straight as possible.

Please note that while we are describing these exercises very quickly on the written page, we encourage you to take the time to put the book aside and actually perform the tonings. The vital essence of insights will come from being in the experience of the sounds, not merely reading about them.

Exercise: Focused Humming

Begin by making a simple humming sound. Feel free to pick any pitch, but it may be best to start with a comfortable tone in the middle of your vocal register. The goal will be to sustain the *mmm* for the comfortable duration of your breath. Perhaps the only starting suggestion for "correct" humming is to be mindful to remain relaxed. Holding tension blocks resonance. Keep your mouth entirely closed but still relaxed and free of facial tension. You may wish to do two or three yawn/sighs to relax and release tension before continuing.

As you make that *mmm* sound, tune in to where you initially feel the resonance. Common initial areas may be in the throat or upper chest. But perhaps it is somewhere else. There is no right or wrong. The goal of all toning exercises is to explore your own unique resonances.

We will now offer some suggestions to experiment with shifting the resonance to new locations. Take another deep, full breath and begin to hum again. As you sustain the *mmm* tone, begin to subvocalize an *ng* sound (as in the last part of the word *hung*). Take care to keep your lips closed and with the *mmm* remaining constant on the same pitch, just imagine that you are beginning to pronounce the *ng*. Notice how the focus of resonance shifts. For many people, this technique will shift the resonance upward, creating more of a nasal focus in the sinus area.

Now try another shift. Begin to drone the *mmm* as before, but allow yourself to subvocally shape an *ooo* tone (as in the word *go*). Notice how the resonance shifts again. Did you find the focus of energy shifting downward this time?

The next step is to begin playing with pitch. Begin with a midrange *mmm*. Over the course of two to three seconds, let your voice drop down to the lowest pitch you can comfortably sustain. Hold the hum for as long as is comfortable. Remain in silence for a few seconds and then repeat the sequence two more times. What did you notice? Did you feel the focus of your humming resonance shifting lower into the body?

Now try the opposite pitch shift. Beginning with a midrange hum, let your pitch shift upward in a similar fashion as above until you reach the highest pitch you can comfortably sustain. Remain in silence for a few seconds and then repeat the upward pitch shift two more times. Continue to take that silent space between tones. What was the experience this time? Perhaps an upward shift in the resonance of your hum?

To take things a little further, let's now add the element of conscious focus. While simply shifting the pitch of your hum may spontaneously target your sound to new areas, the addition of intention often adds a powerful synergy. Try it for yourself. First bring your attention to the base of your spine. Concentrate on the area for a few seconds before beginning your hum. Do three full-breath, low-pitch hums while maintaining your focus on this lower center. Pause for a moment of silence. Now shift your attention to the area of your sternum and repeat the same sequence of three hums on a midrange pitch. Pause for a moment to see how you feel. Finally, shift your attention to the top of your head. Repeat the sequence of three hums on your highest comfortable pitch.

What did you notice? Did the shift in the focus of your attention seem to enhance the targeting of the resonance of your hums?

When you are doing the humming experiments, you will likely find it worthwhile to perform each suggested exercise for a longer period of time. But it does not have to be too demanding at first. A session of five to ten minutes may well be a good starting point. After which, take a period of at least several minutes to sit in silent meditation.

Exercise: Exploring Internal Resonance via Humming

We will now focus on tracking the resonance of the hum as it shifts through your body. Begin by humming again on your lowest pitch. Allow a few seconds for the resonance of the hum to set into place and take a quick mental snapshot of where you first feel it. Then begin slowly raising the pitch higher and higher. Hum and allow the hum to drift upward until you hit your highest comfortable pitch.

Track with your consciousness where the sound resonates. It's highly likely that you will begin by feeling the hum lower in your body. As your pitch rises, the feeling of resonance will typically shift upward through the body, eventually ending up in the head as you reach your highest pitch. Note that it may take a little bit of practice to achieve a smooth, steady flow from your lowest pitch to your highest in one breath. If you have any initial difficulty—do not worry! Just keep trying it in a relaxed fashion, and you will get it within a few moments.

Now that we have experimented with the pure pitch of the hum, let's add the element of focused intention. Begin again with the deepest pitched *hum* sound you can make. But this time, make the sound with the intention that you will feel it at the base of your spine. After you have this sense, slowly raise both the pitch along with the focus of your consciousness and intention simultaneously. Feel the sound rise along your spine as the pitch gets higher and higher. When you reach the highest hum that you can make, feel the focus of the pitch end at the top of your head. If possible, do this exercise in one fluid tone, lasting the full duration of your longest comfortable breath. Repeat the same exercise two more times, and then stop for a few minutes to honor the silence and take note of any energetic resonances that may continue in the space after the sounding. What do you notice?

After a few minutes, repeat the exercise in reverse. This time begin with the highest pitched hum at the top of your head and end with the lowest pitched sound at the base of your spine. As before, there will be natural resonances that occur in the different parts of your physical anatomy simply due to the shifting pitch. But take special note how the resonance of the sound may be enhanced through the focus of your intention. Repeat the descending hum two more times, and then take a few moments of silent meditation. What did you notice this time?

Exercise: Consciously Directed Humming

After you feel comfortable with the previous humming exercises, let's evolve to yet another experiment. For maximum effect, it would be advisable to perform the humming sessions described above several times, ideally with practice sessions on different days.

For this humming session, begin on a comfortable pitch in the middle of your vocal range. Do a hum for the duration of three full breaths just to begin to feel yourself becoming centered and aligned through sound. Next, in the same fashion as described in the latter part of the previous exercise, bring your attention to the base of your spine. This time, simply focus your intention. Leave the pitch of your hum the same.

As you continue to hum on the continuous pitch, begin to shift your attention upward. Trace the full length of your spine with your attention only while remaining on the same pitch. Repeat this exercise two more times, and then rest in a few moments of silence.

What did you notice this time? Did you notice a shift in the resonance of the hum even though your pitch remained the same? Now repeat the variation of the exercise starting with your focus beginning at the crown of your head. Sustain that same midrange hum and guide your attention downward from the top of your head to the base of your spine. Remain in a state of silence for several minutes afterward.

After you have finished the tonings, take a little time to compare the experience of this new technique to the previous sessions. Did you feel a distinct shift in resonances even though the pitch of your hum remained the same? While it's possible that the sensation may have been subtler this time, more like an intuitive energetic "click" than a distinct physical resonance, with continued practice you will note more sensitivity in your ability to direct a tone anywhere simply via the shift in the focus of your attention.

How is this possible? First of all, recall the fact that the human body consists of over 60 percent water. Now imagine throwing a stone into a small children's wading pool. The ripples from the impact will flow throughout the contained body of water. In a similar fashion, any sound that you make will ripple and resonate throughout the body. Water is one of the best and most efficient conductors of sound! Any sound will potentially reach everywhere in the body, and the simple shift in your awareness will heighten the sensation of this fact.

Final Thoughts about Humming

After you have worked though this last sequence, try the variation of humming with your ears closed. Stick your fingers lightly into your ears so that all outside sound is blocked. Begin humming and notice if your experience is different or perhaps even enhanced. Repeat all of the above humming sequences with closed ears, focusing only on the internal resonances. Try making the quietest hum possible and take note that even though the outward sound you are projecting may be barely audible, the internal resonances may be very potent.

This last fact is another reason why the hum may well be the most useful form of therapeutic toning. You can hum anywhere, and if you are in an environment where there is even the slightest bit of background noise—no one will hear you! The hum is always at your disposal as a subtle, yet profoundly powerful, vocal toning tool for transformation and energetic balancing through sound.

Toning Approach Two: Open Voiced Vocal Toning

Now that we have been introduced to the internal resonances produced by humming, it's time to take the first steps into open voiced vocal toning. If you do not have a singing or a voice training background, keep in mind that, as with any new practice, there will be a learning curve to go through. Be gentle with yourself, and be mindful to never strain when doing all of these exercises for the first time.

Although toning is a simple practice that does not require the more technical demands and training of performance singing, remember that the voice box consists of a set of muscles that may require a certain period of time to "get in shape" before you can accomplish everything that you want to with your toning. Consider it to be like beginning a new form of physical exercise. Do your practice sessions in comfortable, measured increments, and you may be surprised how quickly your voice develops.

This next exercise will borrow a common warm-up practice from singing—the vocal siren. We have already done a version of this exercise in the humming section above; we are now simply going to adapt it to an open voiced tone. Described simply, this technique consists of starting on the lowest pitch that you can comfortably hit and allowing the pitch to glide up smoothly to the highest pitch you can sound without strain. And then perform the reverse, starting from your highest pitch sliding down to the lowest.

It is recommended that you begin every day's toning session with a few vocal sirens, just to help relax and loosen up the voice.

As we proceed with the sirening exercise, you may find it useful to be mindful about breath control. In a previous session, we worked with counting as a technique to help regulate the breath. That approach can still be applied now that we are making more open voiced sounds. For example, you may begin by inhaling to a count of four and then sounding to a count of four. If you wish to work on lengthening your tones, experiment with all of the combinations and ratios discussed in the Exhale Breath Practice exercise.

However, now that we are beginning to actually vocalize, some elements of breath regulation should be taken into consideration. Once again, there are some common elements with performance singing, but also some major differences. As with singing, one needs to release enough breath to charge your sounding with enough energy to achieve whatever volume is desired. But one should only release enough breath to support the tone adequately. Not releasing enough air will result in no sound. And releasing too much will cause you to waste air needlessly.

Try the following exercise to create greater awareness of your breath flow. Take a deep full inhale. While exhaling, add a gentle hissing sound to the out breath. Make the first round like a light whisper. Make the sound for as long as you can sustain the tone at a consistent volume. Then, make the hissing sound as loudly as possible. Note how much more breath pressure is required to sustain the louder tone. The duration was probably much shorter due to the fact that you were releasing more air. Next, try a volume at a medium level between the two extremes. After you have a sense of a comfortable midrange pressure, once again try sustaining the tone in the same fashion as the breath counting exercises in the exhalation section.

The goal is to keep the hissing sound even and consistent through the duration. As you begin to attempt the longer breath ratios, you will get a sense of how to pace the timing of your breath release to support your tone consistently. Practice this method with patience! Performance vocalists spend their whole careers working with the subtleties of breath control. Advanced training is not required for vocal toning, but you may wish to work with this practice from time to time. The goal is simply to be able to hold your tones for a reasonable amount of time in order to achieve the desired effects.

Exercise: Vocal Siren

We discussed the basic method of the siren on page 128. Now try it for yourself. Begin toning the lowest pitch you can comfortably sustain. Hold it for a few seconds, and then concentrate on raising your pitch smoothly upward until you reach the highest note you can comfortably hit. Note that it may take a few tries to begin to achieve a smooth sweep. The considerations about breath control apply here as well. But relax and have fun with this practice! There should be no judgments here about how well you are doing it. The main initial goal is to loosen up and begin to let your voice flow freely.

Try the upward sweep a few times, and then reverse the direction. Start at your highest pitch, and let your voice siren downward to your lowest note. Does this sequence feel different from the previous approach?

Do the descending approach a few times, and then try doing up and down in one breath. This one is a little trickier and will require a little more attention to breath flow awareness. But you will get it! Try doing the up and down sequence in the longest breath you can comfortably release, and then try doing up and down in quick sweeps. This move can be one of the better vocal warm-ups for the toning sessions later. Keep playing with the sirening technique, and invent your own variations. For example, mix the up and down in one breath approach with a quick up siren followed by a quick down siren on your next breath.

Exercise: Immersion into Sound, Bringing It All Together

Now that we have been introduced to some aspects of listening, breath, and toning, we will next combine everything previously discussed into a new meditative experience. This meditation will also combine elements from the previous chapters on listening and shamanic practitioner techniques. The exercises from these earlier chapters suggested sonic journeys on both inner and outer sounds. We will now add a very powerful new component—the energy of your own self-created vocal toning sounds. The goal here will be to explore the progression from silence into sound and back to silence. Tune in to the transition between each state, and note any changes you may experience within yourself. Also note how your relationship with your environment may shift as a result of your sounds. Do you believe that it is possible to create shifts and changes in your environment through your sounds?

Begin today's experience by sitting in a comfortable position. Plant your feet on the floor, and make sure that your back is straight with your spine erect. If you are familiar with any particular meditation posture or asana, feel free to assume that position. At a later time, you may also wish to try this meditation lying down, but for now, please begin with an upright posture.

Next, begin taking some deep, full breaths, as you have already been practicing. Inhale to a slow count of eight, hold your breath for a few seconds, and then release the air with a groaning sigh. As you sigh on the exhale, imagine that you are releasing all tension you may be holding. Repeat this sequence several times until you feel a pleasant sensation of relaxation.

Now bring your attention back to your breath. Breathe in an easy, relaxed, even ratio. As you breathe in and out, begin to open your listening awareness, and tune in to the sounds that surround you in whatever environment you may be practicing in. Spend a few moments breathing and listening. Let your attention first drift to the sounds closest to you, and then gradually expand to the most distant sounds you can hear. After a few moments, call your attention back to your immediate surroundings.

After you establish a sense of yourself in your space, begin to add some sound to your breath. Begin by adding a whispering *sss* on the inhale and a breathy *hhaaa* sound on the exhale.

As you begin this gentle sounding, listen to the way that these quiet sounds blend with the ambient sounds of your environment. Good. Now slowly shift to a gentle humming sound at a midrange pitch. Feel the vibrations of your hum, both within your body and how your sounds emanate out into your environment. Continue humming for a few moments. As you do so, feel free to play with your pitch. Try sirening higher and lower within a gentle, comfortable range, and note any differences you may feel.

As you proceed, slowly increase the volume of your hum, and when it feels right to do so, let your sound shift to an open voiced tone. Try using the *aahhh* sound at first. Tone at a comfortable pitch in the middle of your vocal register. As you tone, feel free to play with any of the breath and toning ratios we have previously discussed. But don't be too concerned with counting and measuring. The goal with this exercise is to freely immerse yourself in the pure experience of freely making sound.

After a few moments, begin to let your voice shift to different pitches, sirening up and down in whatever fashion seems most appropriate. You may be surprised to find that your toning begins to take on a life of its own, with your voice spontaneously shifting to different pitches, and perhaps even beginning to form various types of melodies. Let yourself go, and explore where your self-created sound current wishes to take you at this time. It is even possible that you may receive songs of power, such as the ones gifted to shamans during their journeying experiences. If so, you should do your best to remember them, for they will continue to yield new insights and take on more powerful personal resonance as you continue to work with them in the future.

Let your voice play in this fashion for as long as it feels appropriate. But tone for at least several minutes. When you feel that you have completed this part of the experience, shift your sounding back to the humming tone. Hum for a few minutes, letting your volume fade back down to a quiet, internally focused resonance. And then shift to the gentle whispering sounds that we began with, slowly fading your audible sound back to pure breathing as you return your focus to listening to the surrounding ambient sounds of your environment.

Remain in silent meditation for whatever amount of time seems appropriate. After you have returned to your normal state of consciousness, take note of any experiences that may result from this exercise. Do you feel different? More relaxed? Balanced? More in tune with your surroundings? Does the space around you seem different? Brighter? Charged with any different sort of energy? Record any insights into your journal, if it feels appropriate to do so.

Natural Spontaneous Vocal Toning

Before we move on to discuss approaches for toning various targeted subtle energy centers in the next chapters, we would like to consider a very powerful, primal method for tapping into the body's innate energies. This approach involves the natural tones that we make spontaneously in response to various sensations or emotions. We have all been doing this our entire lives. For example, think of a time when you stubbed your toe. What did you do? It's likely that you immediately burst out with an *ow* sound or other spontaneous expression of pain.

On the other side of the coin, have you ever had some kind of accident and tried to not make a sound? It's likely that the experience was even more unpleasant without that release. These spontaneous natural expressions are intuitive forms of toning that arise from our body's innate intelligence. In this case, that vocal sound actually serves to release endorphins that help reduce and balance pain. Natural toning is one of the ways in which our bodies tap into our internal pharmacy of chemicals via sound.

There are many insights to be gleaned from contemplating and then practicing natural body sounds in a mindful fashion. We will simply point out a few in the following pages. But the best classroom is the world. Set an intention to listen to the sounds that people make in response to various sources of stimulation. Be mindful of the sounds you make in various situations and in response to various feelings. These sounds are deeply revealing and some of the most potent energy-shifting sounds possible. They can help you tap into a vast nonverbal language of expression that can be much more powerful than the "who, what, when, and where" stories that we concoct via ordinary speech. The language of direct body energy toning is pure and primal—free of the distortions and misrepresentations than can often be constructed with words. Understanding of the natural body sounds can open the gateway to a powerful method of working directly with the energy and emotional bodies that cannot be equaled by intellectually contrived systems.

There are many examples of spontaneous involuntary toning. Possible articulations include sobbing and wailing as expressions of sorrow or grief or sighs or moans as expressions of relief or ecstasy. Our language is rich with words that depict toning. Phrases such as yawning, groaning, whining, sighing, and grunting are all good examples. And this list is just a start. A bit of reflection could yield many more.

Humans are naturally using toning techniques to express, balance, and regulate energy all the time. The common element is that all of these forms of unconscious toning are autonomic. They happen without conscious contrivance, and the process behind them is often such that they couldn't be stopped even if you consciously tried. Have you ever felt an emotion build up so much you wanted to scream? That desire comes from a source of understanding rooted in your body's innate intelligence that sounding is a means of energy release and transfer.

To set the stage for deeper insights, take the suggestion to listen to the world around you. That mindful listening can serve as your main source of initiation in this realm. In particular, listen to infants and young children. In his years of facilitating the Healing Sounds Correspondence Course, Alec has often been asked, "How can children be introduced to toning practices?" That's an interesting topic, but, in fact, there may well be more to be learned from children, for children often have a natural freedom and uninhibited playfulness with sound. During the process of maturing to adulthood, many people lose this natural spontaneity and become much more shut down in their avenues of sonic expression. There is no judgment here; we have all been subject to this process. But the mission is to become mindful of any inhibitions that we have allowed ourselves to become programmed into and reclaim our natural birthright of freedom of expression via sound. The best way to understand the natural toning sounds is to become like a little child, free to express and playfully ride on the currents of sound courageously, detached from worry about judgments.

The Power of Laughter

All of the forms of primal expression can be adapted into powerful toning practices to work with fundamental body energies and deep emotions. Yet it is not necessary to wait until they are triggered by events outside of your control. It's possible to tap into the related energies via consciously directed cultivation. For our sample practice, we will use the sound of laughter. A similar process could be evoked via any of the tones on the list above, such as groaning or sobbing, but laughter is certainly more pleasant. There may be a lot of deep truth in the popular saying "Laughter is the best medicine!"

Laughter should be mentioned early in any conversation about the power of sound to heal, for it is definitely one of the most powerful healing tones we have available to us. Everyone has experienced the uplifting power of laughing. Laughter at its highest form is a cathartic release. Laughter is a form of unconscious toning. It is universal beyond culture or upbringing. Think about the last time you had a deep laugh. The build up of energy, often felt in the heart center, that spontaneously erupts into sound. Your chest vibrates with the resonance of the sound. The autonomic nature of laughter is formidable. Have you ever tried to stifle a laugh? It's quite difficult. The energy wants to be released. You feel an emotion of joy and humor and automatically express this energy through the sound of laughter. It is pure, joyous energy transmission via sound, usually accompanied with a smile. Often after a great fit of laughter, we will say, "I needed that." The laughter makes us feel lighter because it releases tension. So laughter by its very nature puts us into the relaxed and happy state ideal for recovery and healing.

Laughter is also a means by which to bring people together. It can dissolve barriers. Our friend, the master of laughter and healing, Laraaji Nadabrahmananda likes to quote Victor Borge's statement that "laughter is the shortest distance between two people." When we laugh together we feel an instant and deep rapport. We are resonating with one another with sound created from a place of happiness. We can also consciously evoke laughter as a form of toning. The interesting thing is if you begin to consciously create laughter it will often flow freely into genuine laughter.

Exercise: Laughter Toning

Find a space to make some tones. You might feel self-conscious when doing this exercise. After all, you'll be laughing with yourself. It's silly, and that's okay. In fact, that's part of the exercise. Embrace your inner silliness. Have fun, be playful. Be like a little child in a state of free play with sound! It's been said that play is the spontaneous exploration of sensation. That's the goal of the following exercise. Simply allow yourself to flow the feelings evoked by the sensation of laughter.

Take a deep breath and release it with a sigh. Take another breath and release it with a gentle chuckle. Make whatever laughing sound is natural for you. Continue breathing naturally and making gentle chuckling laughs. Check yourself out—are you smiling? After a minute, expand into deeper laughs. Is the laughter flowing more easily now? Do you find your-self making spontaneous laughter tones, or as it is more commonly known, laughing?

Once you have finished laughing, take a few moments to reset. Check to see if you feel any different. Take note of where you felt the laughter resonating in you. Now you will tone specific laughter tones. See if they are different from your natural laughter tones.

First we will work with the *ha* sound. Breathe in naturally and exhale with a *ha* tone. The *ha* will usu-ally resonate in the upper chest, but notice where it resonates for you. Continue breathing and making *ha* sounds. Try modulating your pitch, making higher and lower *ha* sounds. Notice if changing the pitch on the sound changes where it resonates in you.

Next we will work with the *ho* sound. Imagine yourself becoming the sonic Santa Claus, taking a deep breath and releasing with a deep *ho, ho, ho*. Feel where the sound resonates. How is it different from the *ha* tone? Try to modulate the pitch of the tones. Typically the *ho* resonates in the belly; see if this is true for you.

Finally we will work with the *he* sound. Take a breath and release with a series of *he* tones. Usually *he* will resonate in the head and come out naturally at a higher pitch; check to see if this is true for you. Then change the pitch of your tones, and feel if there is any change in where the sound resonates.

Try alternating between the three tones by making a *ha, ho, he* series. Then try *he, ho, ha*. Notice how the different combinations resonate in your body. Do you feel energy moving around your body as you alternate between the tones? See if you can move the resonance up the body. A suggested series for this would be starting with *ho*, then *ha*, then *he*. Then see if you can move the resonance down your body; a suggested series for this would be *he*, then *ha*, then *ho*.

This exercise shows us how the naturally occurring laughter tones move sound all across the body. Anytime someone laughs, they are using the toning process to spread and express humor and joy. Now you can see that the naturally occurring healing effects of laughter can be consciously utilized.

Take note of this process, and tap into your creativity to adapt this exercise to various other spontaneous body sounds in other sessions in the future. The simple act of consciously "faking" one of these primal sounds can often quickly evoke the real feeling typically associated with the utterance. Once the process is initiated, the tones can quickly become genuine.

As you experiment with these types of toning exercises, you may find that they can open the gateway to powerful emotional and energetic shifts. As you explore, know that you are practicing in a safe container. Another beautiful thing about the power of self-created sounds is that they only take you to a point where you are capable of absorbing and assimilating any resulting experiences. The ultimate source of the sounds is your own inner guidance or higher self. Your own toning serves as a wise and powerful but gentle guide. And all that is required to take the journey is that initial bit of courage to simply open up and make sounds. The sound current itself will guide you to the most beneficial place for you at this point in time.

Recommended Reading

Chanting: Discovering Spirit in Sound by Robert Gass

The Healing Power of the Human Voice: Mantras, Chants, and Seed Sounds for Health and Harmony by James D'Angelo

The Healing Voice: Traditional & Contemporary Toning, Chanting & Singing by Joy Gardener-Gordon

The Roar of Silence: Healing Powers of Breath, Tone & Music by Don G. Campbell

Toning: The Creative and Healing Power of the Voice by Laurel Elizabeth Keyes

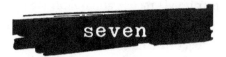
The Energy of the Five Elements

If you want to find the secrets of the universe,
think in terms of energy, frequency, and vibration.

—NIKOLA TESLA

We hope that you began to feel some of the potential for exploring your own energetic resonances via the exercises in the last two chapters. We encourage continued play with the types of toning we've presented. As you continue to do so, you may find continued adaptations and elaborations will come to you. As the gateway to sound begins to open, your own inspirations and intuitions will continue to develop. It's simply a matter of becoming open to it. Now that we have explored some introductory exercises on how to stimulate energy via sound, we'll move on to more specific types of targeted energy work.

Before we proceed, we must admit that the concept of "energy" is somewhat imprecise. We're not talking about bandwidths of energy that can be measured on the electro-magnetic spectrum via meters and quantifiable sensors. The energy under consideration here is more subtle. It may well be more an aspect of consciousness than the measurable physical plane world.

This state of affairs may be the biggest contributing factor to the traditional difficulty energy modalities have had in winning acceptance in currently accepted materialistic scientific arenas. Strides have been made in this sort of endeavor, especially in correlating how subtle energy work affects the currently measurable electromagnetic fields of living organisms, but there is still a long way to go. Perhaps a shift in perspective is necessary. It may well be an issue of proper transduction of these energies. A transducer is basically a device that converts the signal generated by one form of energy to another form of energy. This is a vital concept when considering modulation between different bandwidths of energetic vibration.

For example, imagine trying to measure the energy around you using a radio receiver. That device would be perfectly suited for picking up vibrations in the radio bandwidth, but it will not register the images of television signals. It would be erroneous to believe that television signals do not exist because they can't be received and measured on a radio set. An analogous issue may be present in the gulf between the realms of traditional scientific measurement and subtle energy. The most powerful measuring device may not be some sort of external instrumentation. The full depth of subtle energy may only be properly received by a totally conscious organism.

Conventional physics recognizes only four types of energy: electromagnetism, gravity, and two subatomic forces called the strong and the weak force. Yet various spiritual and wisdom traditions proclaim a much wider spectrum of energies, some rooted in the physical world and some emanating from beyond. Sensitive healers and practitioners of various disciplines often attest to these previously unidentified forms of energy that seem to be capable of interacting with the more easily measurable electromagnetic fields of the body. How is it that they seem to palpably exist in experience, yet be so difficult to validate objectively? The answer may well be rooted in the profound complexity and intricacy of the way our perceptual system processes these energies.

This topic has been masterfully addressed by Dr. Elmer Green of the Menninger Foundation, who performed some of the foundational research in the field of clinical biofeedback. In his book *Beyond Biofeedback*, Dr. Green states:

> ... *[some energies] have not been detected with scientific instruments because these instruments have no parts above the [physical] level. Humans have all the parts and can therefore detect a greater spectrum of energies. Instruments are made of minerals, and lack the transducer components necessary for detection. ... In other words, living beings are coupled to the cosmos better than scientific devices, which are, after all, quite limited tools.15*

---

15. Elmer Green and Alyce Green, *Beyond Biofeedback* (New York: Delacorte Press, 1977), 304.

But it's not necessary to argue about whether or not various subtle energies are "real." We can all experience their effects even without complete understanding of their ultimate nature. In a similar sense, the fundamental natures of commonly accepted energies such as electricity and magnetism are not completely understood. Yet we all benefit from utilizing certain aspects of how these energies behave and by harnessing them in practical ways. Similar rewards may be gleaned from practical, experiential work with subtle energy modalities.

Which brings us back to sound. No one would dispute that sound exists! The study of sound can serve to open the gateway to understanding more subtle octaves of vibration. In a significant sense, at least metaphorically, sound can be thought of as a form of transducer. The energy of sound forms a palpable bridge between the subtle realms and the world of physical manifestation. Sound contributes to a unified field of energy that connects us all. As we have already noted, the entireties of our bodies are emanating sounds. These sounds pulsate from us and create energy fields. All things create these energy fields of sound. So as we move throughout the world, our energy fields are mixing with the fields all around us. Not only are these fields mixing, but through the processes of resonance and entrainment they are affecting each other.

This contemplation of the interaction of energy fields can yield rich rewards. But it can be overwhelmingly mysterious—how can one begin to understand these subtle phenomena? As with our general philosophy regarding sound, direct experience may be the best teacher. And fortunately, the gateway to grasping esoteric concepts can often be opened by contemplating common, everyday events.

To begin, think about the general flow of a typical day. For instance, have you ever woken up and felt you're going very slowly? In this case your internal vibrational patterns are going very slowly. Your natural resonance is slowed, due in part to your environment and the emergence from the slower brain wave and physiological rhythms of sleep. Then when you go outside, you feel the immediate jerk of the sped-up world around you, everything seems to be going very fast. This is because the world around you is operating at a faster vibratory rate. This can be quite jarring at first, because it is an example of your energy fields and those around you being in a slight state of dissonance. Then, in time, as your internal rates speed up to match your surroundings, everything doesn't seem so fast; it just seems normal. This feeling of coming up to speed is the result of your natural resonances entraining with the world around you.

So our own internal vibratory rates are in a state of flux. They vary from slow to very fast within short timespans. This is a good thing. We want to be fluid, flexible beings capable of adapting to various stimuli. Sometimes you can sense when someone's vibratory rate is stuck in a particular range; for instance, when someone seems to always be in a rush and very fiery in all their interactions, they may be stagnating in high-frequency energy fields. On the other end of the spectrum, some people are stuck in very slow vibratory patterns, and they may feel overwhelmed when faced with fast tempo energy fields. This ability to shift our own vibrational rates, to shift frequencies, may well be one of the master skills to be gained for studying subtle energy via sound.

What Are the Five Elements?

A very useful model for understanding vibratory energy is the philosophy of the five elements. The model relates the vibratory rates to the primal elements earth, water, fire, air, and ether. This elemental system has a venerable history and provides a powerful framework for conceptualizing and relating to the fundamental manifestations, flows, and states of basic energy. Note that the five elements philosophy does not refer to physical or chemical compounds as defined on the periodic table of elements in more conventional science, but rather to more metaphorical manifestations of energetic principles. In this sense, the system is more poetically precise. It provides more expansive definitions of energetic processes that also include qualities of consciousness and related modes of being and perception. The inclusion of these dynamics makes it aptly suited to applications in subtle energy work.

The earliest known expression of the five elements cosmology was formulated in the school of classical Indian philosophy known as Samkhya. The primary doctrines of this attempt to explain the origins of the universe and all its beings were formalized by the philosopher Kapila some 2,500 years ago. The revelations of Samkhya have been far reaching and have stood the test of time! The insights of Samkhya have influenced Buddhist metaphysical thought, the cosmological speculations of the pre-Socratic Greek philosophers, and have continued to modern times via the medieval European alchemical traditions into currently active esoteric schools.

Certain contemporary systems of energy work, such as the Polarity Therapy of Randolph Stone, are also deeply rooted in the five elements philosophy. The five element classifications may have been the original system of psychological categorization. Esoteric disciplines and realms of study such as astrology and tarot have been informed by the profound psychological insights stemming from the contemplation of these fundamental elements.

Samkhya offers a rich and detailed cosmology. We will only offer a thumbnail sketch in order to set the foundation for practical working with sound. But the root of the Samkhya outlook is highly significant to our ongoing theme. In his work *Magical Tattwas: A Complete System of Self-Development*, Dr. Jonn Mumford describes the highest level of reality in the Samkhya outlook as follows:

> *Pure, undifferentiated consciousness (Purusha) has always existed. Consciousness was without beginning and without end, eternally radiating through limitless reaches of space and eons of time. Consciousness reflects and expresses itself through an opposite principle, a "consort": Energy (Prakit).*16

So here at the very root of the philosophy we have a profound insight. Even though consciousness and energy are delineated from one other, the synergistic dynamic between them forms an inseparable unity from which the rest of manifestation blossoms. As Mumford goes on to note, consciousness "witnesses" and energy "dynamises." But perhaps

---

16. Jonn Mumford, *Magical Tattwas: A Complete System for Self-Development* (St. Paul, MN: Llewellyn Publications, 1997), 1.

it would be more accurate to state that consciousness directs and energy expresses? Consciousness, in and of itself, has no force to influence, but without the guidance of consciousness, energy is chaotic and lacking direction. The weave and interplay between the two fundamental cosmic aspects of consciousness and energy proceed to shift through various gradients of vibrational rates to ultimately manifest as physical matter. So here at the root of the profound philosophy of Samkhya we have an echoing of the outlook expressed by Dr. Elmer Green: energy and consciousness are intertwined. The subtle energies of the universe will never be measurable independently, but must be understood in the context of interaction with consciousness and as manifestations of states of consciousness.

The Basics of the Five Elements

Discussion of the five elements could easily become very complex and intricate. For indeed, if they represent the five divisions of the infinite expressions of energy in the universe, then each elemental category would be endless in and of itself. We'll simply offer some starting associations below. As you work with the elements, you will likely be initiated into even more dimensions and associations.

On the most basic practical levels, each of the five elements can be correlated with certain speeds of vibration, certain psychological states, and certain behavioral tendencies. They are also linked with particular regions of the body. In this sense, parallels may be drawn with other models of designating energy centers, such as the chakra system (which we will address in chapter 9). But we believe it is useful to consider the elemental centers separately at first.

We will also suggest a system of symbols that can be visualized in conjunction with the five element centers. These images are known as *tattwas*. The tattwa symbols have their roots in the Samkhya tradition and also figure prominently in influential Western esoteric systems of self-development. These tattwa symbols have a charge of psychic energy to them, or morphic resonance, which may also inspire additional insights and inspirations when visualized along with the corresponding tones we will discuss below.

Earth Element

Tattwa Symbol: A yellow square
Location on Body: The base of the spine and lower back, the bottom of the trunk, the legs, and feet

Tattwa Symbol, Square

The earth element could be conceived of as the densest and slowest vibratory rate. It embodies the qualities of groundedness and literal connection to the physical planet Earth. It is important that all energy workings end with a form of grounding, or rooting energies back into the earth. Earth is the source of rootedness and stability. We walk on the earth, we build our homes on the earth, and the food that provides our physical nourishment grows out of the earth.

The earth serves as the foundation for all other elements. In the emotional realm, earth contributes to our sense of security. There could also be associations with practicality, reliability, and common sense, along the lines of the old expression "he has his feet on the ground." Work fueled by the earth energy may be characterized as slow methodical activity, physical presence, attention to detail, and awareness of the physical plane. In terms of vibrational patterns, earth could be expressed by slow, deep pulsing patterns, like the rhythm of a relaxed heartbeat.

Water Element

Tattwa Symbol: A silver crescent
Location on Body: Genitals up through the navel region

Tattwa Symbol, Crescent

On the basic level, the water element can be characterized by the associations one would intuitively connect with it—fluidity and flow. These qualities are also closely related to psychological adaptability and openness to change. Water takes the shape of any container it is poured into. It is formless, yet it can take any shape.

Water could also be associated with persistence. Water is the softest substance, yet it can overcome the hardest. The steady drip of water can erode the hardest rock. Water is related to sensitivity to the flow of feelings of emotion. It's also related to the qualities of intuition and empathy and the energies of sexuality and creativity. Water represents a midrange vibratory rate. It is characterized by calmness and going with the flow. Water would be best expressed by gentle, flowing, fluid rhythms.

Fire Element

Tattwa Symbol: A red upward pointing triangle
Location on Body: The solar plexus (navel up to the bottom of the sternum)

Tattwa Symbol, Triangle

Fire is the third element. It represents a faster vibratory rate with a more energized expression. It is characterized by action, activity, and direct expression. Fire can also relate to personal power, will, and charisma. Fire is an expanding energy that contributes to drive and direct, forward momentum. The confidence to take action is fueled by the fire element. The power of fire can also transmute and purify stagnant or stuck qualities of other element bandwidths. Fire is characterized by sharp staccato, punctuating rhythms, typically at moderately fast to fast tempos.

Air Element

Tattwa Symbol: A blue circle

Location on Body: Heart area (bottom to top of rib cage)

Tattwa Symbol, Circle

Air is the most ethereal of the primary four elements. It represents the fastest vibratory rate. Air is typically a more mental plane energy, fueling the rational mind and intellect. When someone is vibrating in the air element, they are less concerned with the physical plane events around them and more projected into their quick-moving thought processes. Air movement is light, expansive, buoyant, and fast-paced. It can also contribute to energized momentum, but in a less intense way than the fire element. The sound of air is fast-paced, quickly modulating tones. Think of a strong wind whistling through the treetops.

Ether Element

Tattwa Symbol: An indigo oval
Location on Body: Throat

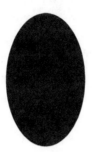

Tattwa Symbol, Oval

The fifth and final element is ether. Ether is considered the highest element, yet it is not really an element at all. Ether is space. Ether contains all four of the previous elements. It is the source from which they all emanate and the destination that they return to after their energy is harmoniously expressed. Ether is the void. However, ether is not a void of emptiness, but rather a pregnant field charged with all possibilities. It is the silent space prior to all manifestation.

Ether relates directly to sound and hearing. The fact that ether is centered at the throat is also thought provoking, for the voice can express the qualities of any of the lower four elements. The sound of ether is silence, yet it's a type of silence beyond the realm of physical plane sound. It could be thought of as a noiseless sound beyond the silence. Ether could also be related to the concepts of the *nada* or *shabda* currents in the sonic yoga traditions.

It is interesting to note that we often use descriptive words related to the elements in daily life to describe people vibrating at particular rates. For example, people are often described as fiery or airy, so the system is already commonly used, just not with the frequency equivalents in mind. No one rate is better than the others. They are all useful in their own particular ways. They have strengths and weaknesses, and they have ideal times for resonance. The key to their ideal existence is a balance between them and an easy transition from one to another.

While we naturally shift through these rhythms as a result of internal processes and external stimuli, we can also directly affect our vibratory rates through conscious thought and use of sound. This can be self-created sound or listening to sound with the specific purpose of shifting our vibratory rate. Many people already utilize this effect without conscious understanding of the vibratory pattern shifting. For instance, many people know that listening to slow, melodic music can help ease them off to sleep. However, if a good workout is your desire, then fast tempo music is in order. In these cases the slow, melodic music would help induce a water or earth element vibratory rate, while the fast tempo music would elicit a fire element vibratory rate.

As noted, shifting through the elements is a natural process. That having been said, people have natural elements they spend far more time in than others, and this is a good thing. This is most likely the vibratory element most resonant with their natural sounds. It only becomes a difficulty when they become locked into vibratory rates and are unable to shift easily (or at all) into others. When this happens, they may feel in conflict with certain aspects of their lives. One of the most palpable examples of this is the clash between parents and teenagers around musical choices. The fast tempo music might well feel comfortable to the teenager's natural resonant element, likely fire, as the hormonal shifts often speed up the nervous system. In juxtaposition, the parent is often vibrating at a slower rate naturally, so their offspring's musical selection seems dissonant and unsettling to their nervous system.

This conflict between different vibratory elements can lead to communication difficulties between people out of sync with one another. Have you ever seen two people arguing over something even though they both agree, but one of them is presenting the information quickly and powerfully while the other is speaking slowly and methodically? Perhaps you've even been in such a situation, where you realize that you agree with the other person—in fact, you're saying the same thing, just in such different ways that you appear to be arguing.

Unfortunately, people operating in different vibratory rates can misinterpret each other. Someone vibrating in the water element might view someone in the fire element as aggressive and rushing, while the person in the fire element might feel they were only being clear and decisive. On the flip side, a person vibrating in the fire element may view a person vibrating in water as lackadaisical, while the water person may feel calm and patient.

To aid in communication, it is helpful to consciously shift your vibratory rate to match the other person. This becomes especially important when trying to help another in a therapeutic fashion. If your vibratory rate is out of resonance with someone you are trying to work on, then you are immediately going to have difficulty connecting with him or her. It is a necessary precursor of effective therapy to match the state of the patient. Much the same as it is a necessary precursor of effective everyday communication. Therefore, working with the five elements can have great practical daily life value above and beyond their applications as subtle energy field balancing techniques.

Bija Mantras and Elements

With this outlook in mind, let us return to practical working with sound. A classic metaphysical aphorism states, "As above, so below." This belief basically posits that the highest levels of ultimate or spiritual reality are mirrored in the "lower" realms of physical manifestation and vice versa. It's a two-way street. Thus, by working with the physical plane energy of sound we can glean insights into the higher orders of reality via our own direct experience.

We will begin with the system of the five primary bija mantras. Before we proceed, note that the term *mantra* more commonly refers to longer phrases or chants. Mantras can be applied for various purposes ranging from devices to enhance meditation to the devotional worship of various deities. We will address these aspects of mantra in a later chapter. Although the bijas are referred to as "mantras," the term is being used here in a more specialized sense. In this case, simply think of them as primal units of sound energy crafted to facilitate attunement to the fundamental essence of their corresponding element. They can be thought of as seed sounds.

The bija syllables do not have literal meanings in and of themselves; their power is based on planting the corresponding energetic seeds into the whole vibratory pattern of one's being. Their purpose is simply to vibrate, invoke, and evoke the power of the element via an intoned sound. In doing so, the mantras can serve to set into motion the vibrations necessary to release any potential energetic blocks, release psychological or physiological blockage within one's being, or perhaps, more positively, serve to activate and initiate new currents of energy conducive to a positive flowering of the element. In a meaningful way, chanting the bijas helps to tune you to the energy of the elements and, via a process of resonance, opens the gateway for the elements to express themselves within your being.

Consider the chanting of the bijas to be a sacred energy working via sound, a type of sacred sound initiation. As with any type of self-development energetic work, it would be ideal to spend a few moments in silent contemplation before practicing the bijas. During this time, set the intention and affirmation that the chanting will bring results to serve your highest purpose at this point in time and that the experience will yield benefits that will harmoniously assist your healing, evolution, and enlightenment in whatever way is most appropriate for you at this point in your development.

In its fullest expression, the system of bija mantras incorporates all of the letters of the Sanskrit alphabet and a number of additional seed syllables. The basic five bijas are written in English as Lam, Vam, Ram, Yam, and Ham. Care should be taken with their pronunciation. We do not wish to suggest judgments about right or wrong ways to do the soundings, but we offer some suggestions based on personal experiences and recommendations from trusted sources.

First of all, the vowel sound in the bijas should not be pronounced as *ah* (as in the words *palm* or *father*), but rather as a soft *uh* sound (as in the words *lung* or *hung*).

In practice, the vowel should also be deemphasized. The primary distinction between the bijas is the initial consonant sound. Other than that, they are all basically the same. Therefore, the main emphasis should be on the first part of the tone when sounding. There are also different ways to end the tone. Many sources teach that the bijas should end with an *mmm* sound, as is implied from the way they are written. Yet we have often found more potent results when substituting a gently nasalized *ng* sound at the end, as in the word *young*.

Indeed, Jonn Mumford recommends this approach in his book *A Chakra Kundalini Handbook*. Mumford notes that in traditional systems of practice, the bijas end with an *mmm* sound when repeated silently, but with an *ng* when intoned audibly. In the spirit of the fluidity of sound, all we can suggest is to feel free to try them both if you feel called to, but we will gently offer preference for the *ng* ending approach. The way in which the final *ng* forms a resonance in the brow, or third eye energy center, seems to magnify the effect of the bijas.

So, to summarize all of the above, we recommend that the bijas be chanted with the main emphasis on the starting consonant, followed by a soft *uh* sound, and end with a nasalized *ng* sound (so that the syllables basically rhyme with the word *young*). The tone should last the full duration of a comfortable breath (as discussed in the toning exercises in the previous chapter). It may take a little bit of practice to establish your own pacing of the component sounds, but, as a general guideline (to use Lam as an example), if your tone lasts for ten seconds, the *lll* sound should extend for five seconds, the *uuh* for one or two seconds, and the *ng* extended for the final three to four seconds.

Exercise: Sounding the Elemental Bijas

Find a comfortable place where you will not be disturbed. The full duration of this exercise may be fifteen to twenty minutes. Take a seated posture with your spine straight. Begin with a few moments of deep breathing. The bijas are traditionally chanted all on one pitch, so take a few seconds to determine a comfortable note. A pitch in the midrange of your vocal register typically works best. As a general rule of thumb, you should chant the bijas basically in the same range as your natural speaking voice. Don't analyze it too much; simply allow yourself to spontaneously chant on a comfortable note.

Before beginning, take a moment to honor and invoke your intention. Acknowledge that you are about to engage in a sacred sound initiation. In your own words, set the affirmation that you will now be harmoniously attuning with the energies of the elements in the way that serves your highest good, and which will assist your evolution and development in the most positive way at this point in time.

Bija Mantra: LAM
First Element: Earth

Bring your attention to the base of your spine and the area encompassing the lower part of your trunk and pelvic floor area. Begin breathing into this area. As you do so, imagine that energy is flowing into the earth center of your body. As you chant the bija Lam, know that this area is becoming balanced and aligned with the resonance of the earth element invoked by the chant. Take a deep breath while continuing to focus on the lower part of your trunk. On the exhale, begin to sound the mantra *lllllll-uuh-nnng* on a comfortable pitch. Let the tone last for the full duration of a comfortable breath. Repeat the Lam mantra seven times. After the last tone, remain in silence for two to three minutes while continuing to focus on and feel your earth center. Continue to breathe energy into this center as you do so.

Bija Mantra: VAM
Second Element: Water

Now bring your attention up to your water center, located in the area between the pubic bone and navel. Begin to breathe energy into this area in the same fashion as with the previous toning. After a couple of minutes, begin to tone the mantra *vvvvvvv-uuh-nnng*. Affirm that as you make the tone, this center is becoming harmonized, balanced, and aligned with the element of water. Repeat the Vam mantra seven times. When you are complete, remain in silence for two to three minutes while continuing to feel the water center. Continue energetic breathing into the area to enhance the activation.

Bija Mantra: RAM
Third Element: Fire

Shift your focus up to the fire center, located in the solar plexus, filling the area between your navel and bottom of the sternum. Begin the energized breathing into this area. When you feel the connection as with the previous centers, start to sound the mantra *rrrrrrr-uuh-nnng*. Repeat the Ram mantra seven times. As you do so, know that this center is becoming activated and charged with the element of fire. After the seventh repetition, repeat the process of meditation and breathing into the fire center as with the previous tones.

Bija Mantra: YAM
Fourth Element: Air

Now bring your attention up to the air center located in the center of the chest. Breathe energy in and out of this area for two to three minutes before beginning to sound the mantra *yyyyyyy-uuh-nnng*. As the sound resonates this area, experience this center balancing and aligning with the element of air. Repeat the Yam mantra seven times. Maintain your focus on this area and perform the energized breathing technique after the last tone.

Bija Mantra: HAM
Fifth Element: Ether

Repeat the process as instructed for the previous four centers. But this time bring your focus up to the throat area and tone the mantra *hhhhhhh-uuh-nnng*. Tone the mantra seven times, and continue focused and energized breathing in and out of your throat area afterwards.

Master Bija Mantra: OM (AUM)
Harmonizing All Elements

After completing the bija mantras for all five elements, you may find it beneficial to perform one final toning. The intention here is to harmoniously align the previous energy centers and circulate their energy throughout the energy fields of your mind, body, and spirit. The mantra we will use here is *om*, which is often recognized as the master bija mantra. In the Hindu tradition, *om* is considered to be the original, primordial creative sound that triggered the manifestation of the universe and all creation. *Om* is the origin of both pure consciousness and all energy. It is commonly pronounced with an *oh* (as in the word *go*) at the beginning and rhyming with the word *home*. Feel free to use that pronunciation if you wish, but for the purpose of this exercise we recommend tweaking it to a fuller spectrum of enunciation.

Indeed, many traditions of Vedic chant advocate that *om* should be pronounced with an *ah* vowel at the beginning (as in the word *father*). We will use that approach here. This pronunciation causes the syllable to make a full sweep through the harmonic spectrum, which enhances its energy activating and balancing effect.

After toning the five element bijas, place your attention on the region between your eyebrows and slightly above (the region often referred to as the third eye area). Breathe a current of energy into this center for a few moments, and then begin to tone *aum*. Begin the mantra with the *ah* vowel as suggested above, sustain through the *oo* (as in *home*), and finally trail off to a humming *mmm* sound. Let each component occupy approximately one-third of your breath, but about halfway through the *mmm* sound, let it transition into a nasalized *nng* sound as with all the previous bijas in this exercise. This technique seems to enhance the targeting of the resonance in the third eye/brow center area.

Tone the *aum* mantra eight times. On the first *aum*, let your awareness remain at the brow center, feeling it as a nexus point that connects all of the elemental centers below. On the second *aum*, continue to feel the vibration in your brow center, but simultaneously let your attention also sweep through all of the previous elemental energy regions. Begin with awareness of the earth center, but let your focus scan upward one at a time through all five element centers evenly. As you do so, imagine that the energy is emanating upward from the earth center forming harmonious connections with all other centers as it rises. Feel that the five elements are becoming synergistically connected in a state of harmonious balance. End with focus in the ether center area.

On the third *aum*, begin with awareness on the ether center and let your awareness flow down through each center successively until you return to earth. As you tone, imagine that the energy is cascading downward from ether, further balancing and aligning each center along the way. Repeat the above sequence, alternating between rising and descending through the elemental energy centers for the next four *aum* tones. On the eighth *aum*, target your focus back on the brow center in the same fashion as the first tone.

After completing the last *aum*, remain in silent meditation for as long as feels appropriate. Feel the energy continue to resonate throughout all of your centers. When you are ready to conclude your experience, shift your focus back down to the earth center. Tone several more Lam mantras in quick succession to ground your experience back to earth and back into the physical body. Make them slightly louder and more forceful than during the main meditation. You may also wish to stand up to move and stretch. Feel your feet and imagine roots of connection from the soles of your feet down into the center of planet Earth. Affirm that you are now fully back in your body, yet still connected with the currents of the five elements.

Exercise: Sounding the Elemental Bijas with Tattwa Visualizations

After you have had the experience with pure sound in the previous exercise, you may wish to try a more advanced variation. This time we will add a visualization component. You will basically repeat the bija tonings as described above, but this time visualize the corresponding tattwa symbols. For best results, try this variation for the first time on a new day.

When you perform the energized breathing before each sounding, imagine the appropriate tattwa symbol shining in each energy center. During the initial period of silent focus before each toning, breathe into each energy center through the image of the symbol. See the symbol getting brighter as you breathe into it, and watch it continue to glow with more radiance as you perform the bijas. See the symbol continue to shine during the silent meditation afterward before shifting your awareness to the next center. This additional extension of the visualization will serve to enhance the continued synergy of the energy of the symbol with the sound you have just created.

For this new experience, simply follow the instructions for the Sounding the Elemental Bijas exercise, but also incorporate the following tattwa symbol visualizations:

Lam Bija/Earth Element: A yellow square
Vam Bija/Water Element: A silver crescent

Ram Bija/Fire Element: An upward pointing equilateral triangle

Yam Bija/Air Element: A blue circle

Ham Bija/Ether Element: An indigo oval

Additional Elemental Bija Variations

Perform the bija toning experience again, but begin with the *aum* tone at the brow center. Then proceed downward to the ether center at the throat and proceed through all centers until you reach earth. Note any differences in your experience of tracking the elements flowing down from above as opposed to emanating upward from below.

After you have experienced the full meditation several times, try a shorter version. The prior experiences with the full-length elemental meditation will likely serve as an anchor, rooting the balancing effects of the bija toning into the energy pattern of your being. After this patterning takes place, you may find that you can still achieve powerful results with a much shorter experience. In this quick tune-up version, tone each elemental bija once, followed by three *aum* sounds to complete the elemental balancing and circulation. Take note if this quick version still evokes similar feelings as the full experience. It may well not be as deep as the extended bija meditations, but it will certainly have convenience value! You can give yourself a quick elemental energy tune-up in a couple of minutes anytime throughout the day. Repetition of this short exercise will have compounded benefits as you become accustomed to making elemental balancing a regular part of your day blended with the flow of your regular activities.

Recommended Reading

Magical Tattwas: A Complete System for Self-Development by Jonn Mumford

Music and Sound in the Healing Arts: An Energy Approach by John Beaulieu

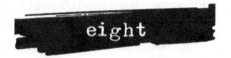
eight

Further Initiations into the Five Elements

The universe has originated from the tattwas (the elements).
All changes in the world of names and form
are changes in the elements. ... The elements are,
O Devi, the main constituents of the universe.
—EXCERPT FROM THE SWARA YOGA SCRIPTURES

Now that we have explored a particular traditional system of tones that work with the five elements in the past chapter, we would like to offer an approach from a completely different perspective. We would encourage continued exploration of the bija mantra exercise. Be sure to try variations, such as doing the tonings at different times of the day. Pay attention to how the variations in your mood and energy state prior to going into the meditation may affect the results of your experience.

Although the bija mantra system is very powerful both in terms of the pure resonances triggered by the sounds and the morphic fields it may help you tap into, it's worth noting that it is only one system. We are all unique vibratory beings, and there is no one system that will be suitable for everyone at all times. Ultimately, any system is merely a model. Any given model is worth studying and experiencing on its own terms, but no one model will ever account for all aspects of a phenomenon. Ultimately, we will again stress the importance of experimentation in your own sonic laboratory.

In that spirit, we will now offer you a series of guided meditations. During these meditations you will imagine yourself present with each of the elements. This will allow you to consciously merge with each element and then find a spontaneous, intuitive sound that represents and resonates with that element for you. In the process, you may well find yourself guided to make a previously learned sound. If so, then that's all fine! That discovery will serve to validate the personal value of the sound, above and beyond merely repeating a sound that was prescribed from some authority.

On the other side of the coin, you may also find yourself guided to make completely different, unexpected tones. Honor these discoveries! These spontaneous connections have the potential to be some of the most powerful personal initiations into sound and vibration.

In the following exercise, know that there is no right or wrong. Allow yourself to engage in free play with the sound current! These sounds will be yours, and there will be no judgments. In the following meditation, you will be working with all five elements. For this first session, we recommend that you use some kind of timer, or at least mentally set your intention, to limit your time at five minutes per element. The goal here is to journey through all five elements in one session and find your own personal elemental tones. Know that you can return to any or all of them to work in further depth at a later time via the same techniques.

Exercise: Guided Imagery Elemental Sound Journeys

To begin, find a space where you can make sound freely. Get into a comfortable posture with your spine straight. Spend a few moments aligning yourself with rhythmic breathing. Then take a deep breath and hold it for a few seconds. Release that breath with a drawn-out sigh. As you do so, feel all tensions release and allow yourself to settle into a deep state of relaxation. Repeat the deep breath with sighing release a few times.

Earth Element Journey

When you are ready, close your eyes. Continue rhythmic breathing for a few moments while imagining that you are breathing in and out through your brow center. Feel a pleasant sensation of relaxation continue to spread throughout your being as your inner vision begins to open. Now imagine a door in front of you. A large yellow square, the tattwa symbol for earth, is painted on this door. In your mind's eye, see yourself getting up to open and walk through this door. As you pass through the doorway, you are transported to an open meadow in the middle of a forest. Walk to the center of this meadow and lie down on the earth.

Feel yourself lying directly atop the earth, nothing between you and the soil below you. It is brown and dry and smells of life. Feel yourself settle into the earth, feel your limbs gently spread and imagine that you have roots that reach down far below the surface. Merge with the earth and feel yourself become one with the fertile soil all around you. As you feel that connection, take a deep breath and release with a sigh. Pause for a moment and invite the energy of earth to sound through you. Then take another breath and release with a sound, whatever tone comes spontaneously as your own personal expression of the earth energy. Spend several minutes sounding this tone, allowing yourself to be an open instrument for any sounds and rhythms that may come through.

When your time is up, offer thanks to the energy of earth and feel yourself disconnect from its energy. See the same doorway that you used to enter the realm of the earth element appear before you again. Pass through that doorway and return to your physical body. Clap your hands three times and announce that this particular journey into the realm of earth is concluded. Begin to move your limbs and stretch your body until you begin to feel fully grounded and present. Take the time to write down the sounds that came to you during your journey. Know that you can continue your communion with the element of earth at any time by sounding these tones or by repeating the journey that initiated the exercise.

Water Element Journey

Give yourself a moment to relax and reset before continuing to the next element. When you are ready, close your eyes. Continue rhythmic breathing for a few moments while imagining that you are breathing in and out through your brow center. Feel a pleasant sensation of relaxation continue to spread throughout your being as your inner vision begins to open. See a door in front of you decorated with a large silver crescent, the tattwa symbol for water. Pass through the door as before, and find yourself transported to a beach.

Walk down to the very edge of the shore and sit down on the damp sand. The air smells of the ocean, salty and clean. Hear the ocean waves crashing in front of you, and let your gaze drift over the rising and falling surf. Feel your spirit merging with the ocean and allow yourself to drift out onto the waters. Feel yourself floating weightlessly, surrounded by the nurturing waters. Imagine that you can expand and connect with all the waters of the world—every river, stream, lake, and waterway. Take a deep breath and release with a sigh. Invite the energy of water to sound through you. Then take another breath and release with a sound, whatever sound comes naturally. Spend several minutes sounding this tone, allowing yourself to be an open instrument for any sounds and rhythms that may come through.

When your time is up, offer thanks to the energy of water and feel yourself disconnect from its energy.

See the same doorway that you used to enter the realm of the water element appear before you again. Pass through that doorway and return to your physical body. Clap your hands three times and announce that this particular journey into the realm of water is concluded. Begin to move your limbs and stretch your body until you begin to feel fully grounded and present. Take the time to write down the sounds that came to you during your journey. Know that you can continue your communion with the element of water at any time by sounding these tones or by repeating the journey that initiated the exercise.

Fire Element Journey

Take another moment to relax and reset. When you are ready, close your eyes. Continue rhythmic breathing for a few moments while imagining that you are breathing in and out through your brow center. Feel a pleasant sensation of relaxation continue to spread throughout your being as your inner vision begins to open. This time you pass through a doorway marked with a red upward pointing triangle, the tattwa symbol for fire.

After passing through the doorway, you find yourself in the midst of a desert. As you walk forward, you come upon a fire pit that is all set up with the makings of a bonfire. See sparks begin to dance about the wood and tinder, quickly spreading into open fire. The flames start low but quickly rise. As the flames rise into a raging blaze, you feel the fire rise within. Smell the smoke;

feel the crackling heat. Realize that the fire before you mirrors the fire rising within you. Again take a deep breath and release with a sigh. Invite the energy of fire to sound through you. Take another breath and release with a sound, whatever sound best expresses the energy of the fire you feel within and without. Spend several minutes sounding this tone, allowing yourself to be an open instrument for any sounds and rhythms that may come through.

When your time is up, offer thanks to the energy of fire and feel yourself disconnect from its energy. See the same doorway that you used to enter the realm of the fire element appear before you again. Pass through that doorway and return to your physical body. Clap your hands three times and announce that this particular journey into the realm of fire is concluded. Begin to move your limbs and stretch your body until you begin to feel fully grounded and present. Take the time to write down the sounds that came to you during your journey. Know that you can continue your communion with the element of fire at any time by sounding these tones or by repeating the journey that initiated the exercise.

Air Element Journey

Take a few moments to relax before preparing yourself for a new journey. When you are ready, close your eyes. Continue rhythmic breathing for a few moments while imagining that you are breathing in and out through your brow center. Feel a pleasant sensation of relaxation continue to spread throughout your being as your inner vision begins to open. This time you will pass through a door decorated with a blue circle, the tattwa symbol for air.

As you pass through the doorway, find yourself transported to the top of a mountain at the height of the world. The sky around you is brilliantly clear, and the air is crisp and clean. Feel the tickle of air on your skin as a gentle breeze begins to blow. Feel the strength of the air build as the gusts grow stronger, quickly building into a stiff wind. Feel the wind wash over you. Taste its rich, pure sweetness. Hear its speed as it whips and changes direction. As you inhale and exhale, realize that the air around you is the same as the air within that fuels your mind and spirit. Once more take a deep breath and release with a sigh. Invite the energy of air to sound through you. Take another breath and release with a sound, whatever sound comes naturally. Spend several minutes sounding this tone, allowing yourself to be an open instrument for any sounds and rhythms that may come through.

When your time is up, offer thanks to the energy of air and feel yourself disconnect from its energy. See the same doorway that you used to enter the realm of the air element appear before you again. Pass through that doorway and return to your physical body. Clap your hands three times and announce that this particular journey into the realm of air is concluded. Begin to move your limbs and stretch your body until you begin to feel fully grounded and present. Take the time to write down the sounds that came to you during your journey. Know that you can continue your communion with the element of air at any time by sounding these tones or by repeating the journey that initiated the exercise.

Ether Element Journey

Prepare yourself as in the previous journeys. When you are ready, close your eyes. Continue rhythmic breathing for a few moments while imagining that you are breathing in and out through your brow center. Feel a pleasant sensation of relaxation continue to spread throughout your being as your inner vision begins to open. Then see a door in front of you marked with an indigo oval, the tattwa element for ether.

As you pass through that portal, imagine that you begin to expand. Feel your being grow into space, expanding beyond the room you are currently in. Continue expanding above and beyond the whole building where you find yourself. Grow to fill the whole yard outside, then your whole neighborhood, then your whole town. Continue until your being expands beyond the boundaries of the entire earth. From there, look out and see the countless stars and galaxies beyond. Imagine that your awareness can continue to expand to touch those distant lights, and beyond.

Now, invite the element of ether to sound through you. Take a deep breath and release with a sound— whatever tone best expresses the vast energy of space. Spend several minutes sounding this tone, allowing yourself to be an open instrument for any sounds and rhythms that may come through. Note that it's possible that this tone may be beyond the range of what you can physically vocalize. If so, then simply imagine the sound. Hear it psychically ringing throughout space and all dimensions, physical and etheric.

When your time is up, offer thanks to the energy of ether and feel yourself disconnect from its energy. Allow your awareness to shrink back down again until you pass through the original doorway and return to your physical body. Clap your hands three times and announce that this particular journey into the realm of ether is concluded. Begin to move your limbs and stretch your body until you begin to feel fully grounded and present. Take the time to write down the sounds that came to you during your journey. Know that you can continue your communion with the element of ether at any time by sounding these tones or by repeating the journey that initiated the exercise.

You have now manifested your own set of elemental sounds. We hope that you enjoyed this experience and will continue to explore your own elemental resonances via these techniques. Know that these sounds may continue to evolve as personal tones of power. These tones that emanate from your own inner guidance, inspiration, and connection with your own higher source can be as valid and potent as any sounds learned from outside authorities, and, in many cases, perhaps more so. This type of exploration can be thought of as another type of sonic shamanism. As noted in a previous chapter, the true source of shamanic power derives from direct contact with other realms of consciousness and energy. Then the task is to bring these experiences back for practical applications on this plane.

When you feel called to do so, return to the sounds you created during this exercise. You may wish to incorporate them into a full-length meditation along the lines of the session we performed with the bija mantras, but instead substituting your own tones. Or you may wish to do separate sessions devoted to single elements one at a time. With a little more practice and familiarity, these tones could be utilized for quick energy tune-ups in the midst of your day to evoke the energy of a desired element to assist with whatever task is at hand. There are many possibilities. As you continue to work with sound, your creativity will continue to blossom and new applications will come to you that are uniquely yours.

Joshua and Alec's Elemental Tone System

To close this chapter, we would like to share an elemental tone system that we created using guided meditation journeying. It is a very simple system that shares some traits with other classical systems. We have shared these tones in group settings, and a high percentage of people have found them to be natural, easy resonances that are simple to learn. But note that the following exercises are only sample suggestions. You could also perform the same applications with your own unique elemental tones.

Here's the system:

Earth Tone: *Uh* as in the word "up."

Water Tone: *Ooo* as in the word "you."

Fire Tone: *Rah* as in the word "raw."

Air Tone: *Ah* as in the word "father."

Ether Tone: The final sound representative of the ether energy is not a pronounced tone like the others. To perform this tone, simply allow air to glide in and out on the breath in a whispering fashion while imagining an expansive sense of space. Make your tone sound like a gentle breeze.

These tones can be used independently or in concert with one another depending on the desired effect. Pay attention to see if there is one energy type you resonate with more strongly and if there is one you find more difficult to resonate. This can be an important clue for you as to which elemental range you spend most of your time in and which you utilize rarely. There are times in our lives when all types of energy are useful. These exercises will allow you to see the power of sound to initiate shift through the elemental energy patterns. To apply these tonings, think of situations where the appropriate elemental energy would be a useful ally.

Exercise: Generating Earth Energy

Earth energy is by its nature grounded and solid. It is detail oriented, ideal for research or study. Earth energy is also perfect for detail-oriented tasks. Earth can be useful to center and relax if you find yourself feeling scattered or in a state where it's difficult to focus. Earth energy can also be useful for concerns related to housing, work, money, partnerships, and connection with one's physical body. For this exercise, you'll be utilizing the earth tone from our system, which is *uh* as in *up*.

To connect with earth energy, find a space in which to make sound. Take a moment to internally scan yourself. How are you feeling? How much energy do you have? Are you tired, or are you energized? It's important to take measure of how you're feeling now so you can notice how the sound affects you. This exercise should be done with the intention of slowing down and creating stability.

Take a deep breath, and release with a sigh. Take another breath and release with a low-pitched *uh* sound for the full length of the exhale. You should make note where the sound resonates within you. Continue to inhale deeply and exhale with an *uh* sound for about a minute. With each repetition, increase the length of the sound. As you sound, bring at least 20 percent of your attention to the soles of your feet to facilitate a feeling of rootedness and connection with the ground below you.

Exercise: Generating Water Energy

Water energy can be very useful in our lives when we are feeling stuck or tense. It is the great fluid energy that allows us to calmly maneuver past obstacles. Water can also be used to stimulate creativity and imagination. Water also assists with the free flow and expression of emotions. Water always wants to flow, and the nature of water is to follow the path of least resistance.

To generate water energy, begin to sound the *ooo* syllable as in the word *you*. Tone in a flowing rhythm with gentle fluctuations in pitch. You may also wish to make gentle rotations of your shoulders and hips as you tone. Feel all tensions in your body begin to release and flow. As you continue to tone, begin to feel your being become more fluid with greater adaptability and sensitivity.

Exercise: Generating Fire Energy

Fire energy can be very important when we need to accomplish a physical task or if we are feeling tired. Fire contributes to energized motivation, personal power, and directness of expression.

To build fire energy, you'll be utilizing the fire tone from our system, which is *rah* as in *raw*. This exercise should be done with the intention of building energy. Take a deep breath and release with a sigh. Place your hand in front of your solar plexus. Now take a deep breath and release with an elongated *rah* sound. Repeat this three times. As you make the sound, imagine smoldering embers deep within you. Now begin to chant the *rah* sound, breathing normally and establishing a rhythmic pulse. Shift the tone into a faster, more percussive rhythm. As you chant, imagine that you are fanning the embers within. As you feel the energy build within you, the embers glow brighter and brighter red, until they burst into flame. You can grow this flame to be as big as you need to fuel the energy for whatever may come.

Exercise: Generating Air Energy

Air can aid mental focus and clarity of thought as well as verbal expression and intellectual pursuits. Air can also contribute to lightness of being and a sense of uplifting expansion. Think of an eagle in flight as it gently and effortlessly soars on the wind currents.

To activate the air element, tone the sound *ah* as in *father*. But let the sound have an almost whispering quality as it gracefully glides on the breath. Modulate the pitch of the tone in quick fluctuations. Think of the wind whistling through the treetops.

Exercise: Generating Ether Energy

The benefits of generating ether energy may be the most elusive to define, but they could well be the most expansively useful. Ether can contribute to an expansion of your awareness, to a more mystical state of being with an enhanced connection with all creation. When you can expand your consciousness above and beyond a narrow focus on daily problems and concerns, you might find that these issues begin to diminish. Ether can also foster connections with the highest and deepest sources of inspiration and enlightenment.

To resonate with ether, breathe in and out in an even rhythm while adding a slight whispering inflection to the voice. The audible sound will be very faint, but as you tone feel the energy of your tone expanding outward. Make sound on both the in breath and out breath. As you tone out, feel that your sound expands to fill the heavens. As you tone in, feel the vastness of the universe flow into you, expanding your boundaries to the infinite. Allow for a few seconds pause between inhalations and exhalations and tune in to the stillness at this point of rest. Feel the pregnant possibility of space and silence, for it is the nothingness out of which all possibilities are born.

And on that note, we will conclude this journey into the realm of the five elements. We hope that these exercises will serve to open the gateway to working with these fundamental energies—to serve as an initiation, if you will. Note that the term "initiation" simply denotes a beginning.

As you continue to work with the elements, many more vistas of insight will open up. The five elements are simple building blocks, yet their evolutions and nuances can be infinitely complex. The dynamic synergy between the basic elements forms the alchemical symphony of all creation and experience. May the resonances of your own sounds serve to attune you to the universal dance of elemental vibrations, both within and without! Now that we have explored general qualities of energy, let us move on to working with even more specific targeted energy centers.

Recommended Reading

Magical Tattwas: A Complete System for Self-Development by
Jonn Mumford

Music and Sound in the Healing Arts: An Energy Approach by
John Beaulieu

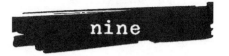

nine

Vocal Toning Part Three

Resonating the Chakras

*We have five senses in which we glory and which we recognize
and celebrate, senses that constitute the sensible world for us.
But there are other senses—secret senses, sixth senses, if you
will—equally vital, but unrecognized, and unlauded.*

—OLIVER SACKS

In the previous chapter, we discussed broad general band-widths of energy categorized by the five elements. We will now tune the focus a little more. We will next concentrate on more specific centers in the energy body known as the chakras and how you can resonate, energize, and balance them with vocal toning practices.

Whereas the five elements represent broader levels of energy classification, the energy centers behave more like structural elements in the pattern of one's energy field, and they can potentially have more direct resonance on one's physical state of being. They could be thought of as a type of energy anatomy. There are a number of different systems and ways of defining the energy centers, but we will first focus on the popular model of the seven chakras.

What are the chakras? They are basically energy centers located vertically along the centerline of the body. The chakras run from the base of the spine up to the crown of the head. The word *chakra* is of Sanskrit origin. The term stems from the root *car*, "to move,"[17] and can basically be translated as *wheel*, *disk*, or *circle*. Chakras are often pictured as moving vortexes or open spinning flowers. One common element in the depiction of chakras is motion. They are not static objects but rather vibrant, pulsating energetic fields. In a fashion analogous to our physical organs, these fields function to facilitate life. In various processes similar to how the heart pumps blood on the physical body level and the liver clears toxins, the chakras serve comparable purposes on higher energetic levels. For our purposes, we will view chakras as anchors and transduction points of energetic flow that connect our individual beings to more subtle body fields of energy. The chakras are like the receiving stations through which broader currents of universal energy, such as the bandwidths expressed by the five elements, are translated into the fields of our mind and body.

The concept of chakras is ancient. The chakras are found in many traditions, including Hindu and Tibetan. Many esoteric and occult mystery schools also describe these energy centers. While the chakras have been incorporated in many spiritual practices, their existence seems to be based not upon

---

17. Leza Lowitz and Reema Datta, *Sacred Sanskrit Words: For Yoga, Chant, and Meditation* (Berkeley, CA: Stone Bridge, 2005), 65.

religion but upon awareness of energy. Indeed, the chakras may be in part co-created by our own awareness in the way that we focus our own consciousness.

This concept is supported by the fact that there are a number of different chakra systems found in various traditions. We will focus primarily on the popular seven chakra model rooted in the Vedic tradition. Yet it's interesting to contemplate that the Tibetan system only defines five chakras. The elaborate energy anatomy system found in Chinese medicine does not emphasize chakras at all! That framework notes three primary energy centers known as *dan tiens*, which are connected by an intricate web of energy pathways called meridians. To further complicate matters, even more new chakra system models are continuing to emerge from various contemporary energy work schools. We have seen systems advocating the existence of eight chakras, thirteen chakras, even up to twenty-one chakras.

What is one to make of this? Which one is "true"? Perhaps the contemplation of sound can yield a clue? The musical octave can be divided up into numerous intervals and scales. These musical divisions vary widely in different cultures and different genres of music. Perhaps in an analogous fashion, the human energy system can also be compartmentalized in a multitude of ways. They can all serve as useful models within their given frameworks depending on the desired results of their practitioners.

However, it's not our purpose here to go into great depth about the particulars of these varying systems. Please see some of the works in the recommended resources list for further information. Our intention for the time being is rather to show how chakras can be useful centers on which to focus and project sound. We have already discussed how sound can activate and create energy fields. If the chakras are really just fluid patterns of energy, then sound can be a potent tool to modulate these energetic structures. In doing so, sound can serve as an invaluable ally to fine-tune the subtle mechanisms by which the chakras transduce universal currents of energy into expression in our own minds, bodies, and spirits.

In various systems, chakras correspond to nerve plexuses, endocrine glands, and body parts. Chakras can also be related to developmental characteristics, levels of consciousness, and archetypal energies, in addition to many other associations. Each chakra carries a unique vibrational resonance, which is dynamically influenced by a range of factors. Chakras are also often correlated with systems of corresponding colors.

Though we too will be offering example of such associations, it's worth noting at the outset that the systems are not perfect. For example, if we say that a chakra has a certain location in the body, note that the energy of the chakra is not limited to being bound to that place. The physical associations may serve merely as convenient labels to allow us to focus on the energy of the chakras. As for colors, if one studies various sources throughout the history of esoteric literature, one will find numerous conflicting colors associated with any given chakra. The most popular contemporary system is to associate the chakras with the "ROY G BIV" rainbow spectrum, which stands for red, orange, yellow, green, blue, indigo, violet. We like this system, but it's worth noting that this particular set of chakra color correspondences has only evolved as an accepted consensus within the last twenty years or so. It can nonetheless serve as a useful practical model for beginning to work with the chakras.

Chakra Balancing

There are seven main chakras. The chakras are transduction points—places where subtle energy from higher planes converts to physical form. The energy from the chakras then becomes denser as it comes into the solidity of the physical body. Frequently, healers who work with subtle energy can detect imbalances before they manifest in the physical body by feeling imbalances in the chakras, for the chakras mediate all energy within, flowing into, and emanating out of the body. Thus by balancing the chakras, imbalances in the physical body will often disappear.

Throughout the various source traditions, there is a common understanding that imbalances in these subtle energy centers leads to distress in the physical and emotional bodies. Ancient healers and shamans would use sound to help realign and balance these energy centers.

There is a feedback loop occurring with the energy of the chakras. The physical body interfaces with this energy and vice versa. Frequently, an imbalance in a chakra will manifest later in the physical body. But it is possible, such as through a traumatic injury, for both the physical body and the chakras to be simultaneously imbalanced. Healing of the physical occurs much more rapidly when the subtle anatomy—particularly the chakras—is aligned after physical injury. Frequency shifting through resonating the chakras allows us to help create balance and alignment within ourselves on physical, mental, emotional, and spiritual levels.

The system we will focus on accounts for seven main chakras, seven spinning balls of energy that are located centrally along the front and back of the body. The following is a brief description of the chakras. Note that the first five chakras are also closely associated with the five elements, and thus all of the attributes discussed in the last chapter pertaining to the five elements could also be applied to their respective chakras.

First Chakra

Root Chakra

The first or "root" chakra is located at the base of the spine or in the perineum region. The Sanskrit term for this chakra is *Muladhara*, which means "root support." The root chakra is involved with the physical process of elimination and the organs that work with that function. It is the chakra associated with the energy of physical security and survival. This chakra is also associated with grounding to the physical plane. The color usually associated with the chakra is red. The elemental quality is earth. A common endocrine gland association is the adrenals.

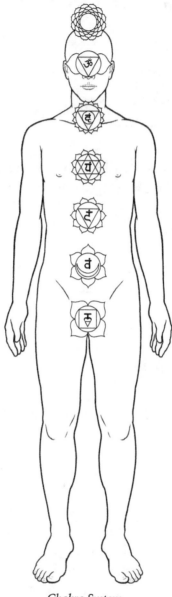

Chakra System

Second Chakra

Sacral Chakra

The second or "sacral" chakra is located midway between the pelvic bone and the navel. The Sanskrit term is *Svadhistana*, meaning "sweet abode of the self." This center is associated with sexual energy, with the reproductive organs, and with much of the life force. It is also the center of creativity. The color for the sacral chakra is orange, and the element is water. Endocrine gland associations are the testes and ovaries.

Third Chakra

Solar Plexus Chakra

The third or "navel" chakra is located in the solar plexus region midway between the navel and the bottom of the rib cage. The Sanskrit term is *Manipura*, meaning "lustrous gem." Its energy is associated with digestion and the digestive organs. It is also associated with personal power. The third chakra is related to passion, power, motivation, the expression of energy, and self-mastery. Its color is yellow, and the element is fire. Possible endocrine gland associations are the pancreas and adrenals.

Fourth Chakra

Heart Chakra

The fourth chakra is known as *Anahata* in Sanskrit, which means "unstruck." It's commonly referred to as the "heart" chakra and is located in the center of the chest between the nipples. On the physical level, it works with the lungs and the heart. On the emotional level, it works with the energy of compassion and love. The color is green, and the associated element is air. An endocrine gland association is the thymus.

Fifth Chakra

Throat Chakra

The fifth or "throat" chakra is located at the throat, at the base of the neck. The Sanskrit term is *Vishuddha*, meaning "purification." It is the chakra that is associated with the process of communication—speech and hearing. The ears are

associated with this chakra, as is, of course, the vocal apparatus. The elemental quality is ether, and the color is blue.
Related endocrine glands are the thyroid and hypothalamus.

Sixth Chakra

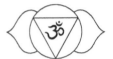

Third Eye Chakra

The sixth or "brow" chakra is *Ajna* in Sanskrit for "perceive
and command," and it is located in the center of the forehead above the eyes. Often called the third eye, it is associated with imagination, intuition, and psychic visions and
abilities. General mental activity and brain function are also
associated with this chakra. The color is indigo. This chakra
transcends the five element qualities attributed to the centers
below, but it could be thought of as the nexus point where
they join into harmonious circulation in one's energy body
field. A common endocrine gland correlation is the pineal.

Seventh Chakra

Crown Chakra

The seventh or "crown" chakra is located at the top of the
head. It is known as the *Sahasrara,* or "thousandfold lotus"

in Sanskrit. The crown is associated with the induction of spiritual energy into the body. The seventh chakra is related to transpersonal consciousness and spiritual awakening. It is said to control every aspect of the body and mind and is associated with full enlightenment and union with the divine. This chakra is normally not fully open in most humans, though pictures of saints and other spiritual beings with halos are depictions of activated crown chakras. This chakra functions as a transduction station through which universal sacred energies resonate into the individual energy field and vice versa. The related endocrine gland is the pituitary—although note that some systems assign the pineal to this center and the pituitary to the third eye.

Balancing the Chakras through Sound

In a nutshell, chakras are energetic structures that transduce or translate energy into our physical form and mental/emotional/psychological beings. They are not things, but rather vortexes of energetic processes or simply energy fields. We have already discussed how sound has powerful abilities to shape, form, and create energy fields. Therefore, the chakras are perfectly suited to being charged, aligned, and balanced via sound.

In reality, there are a multitude of sonic systems one could use to resonate the chakras. However, one approach that manifests in many sources and traditions is the use of vowel sounds to resonate these centers. The power of the vowels is quite extraordinary to contemplate! At first consideration, the vowels may seem commonplace since they are simply part of ordinary speech. Yet the power and sacredness of vowels has been known for thousands of years in both the Eastern and the Western mystery schools.

In Kabbalah, the mystical path of the Hebrew tradition, the vowel sounds are considered the vibrations of heaven. In complementary contrast, the consonants contained the energy of the earth. Via the alchemy between the two, communication between heaven and earth became possible. Certain Kabbalists also believe that the true sacred name of God is actually composed solely of vowel sounds. In Sufism, the mystical path of the Islamic tradition, the power of the vowels and their divine attributes is also understood.

A more contemporary source for the power of the vowels is Edgar Cayce, who was known as the Sleeping Prophet during his activity in the 1920s and 1930s. Cayce would basically go to sleep and channel extraordinary information about healing and esoteric material. On a side note, one of Cayce's striking statements was that "the medicine of the future will be sound." Indeed, we are rapidly approaching this future. In his information, Cayce talked about the priests in ancient Egypt having knowledge of the seven sacred vowel sounds to resonate their energy centers.

Contemplation of the vowels as sacred sounds is not limited to channeled information sources. In his fascinating book *The Mystery of the Seven Vowels*, noted scholar of Western esoteric traditions Joscelyn Godwin offers an overview of the usage of the vowels in various wisdom traditions and spiritual systems. One of his key points relates to how the simple seeming vowels express universal properties pertaining to how sound manifests in our perception. Recall the discussion of harmonics in chapter 1. The vowels, by their nature, express and articulate different harmonics. And in doing so, they also express various ratios and geometry. In contemplating the universal appeal of vowel resonances, Godwin states:

> *Another conclusion to be drawn from the uncon-scious hearing of vowel-resonances is that we must have an inborn familiarity with the harmonic series. Some-where in our perceptive mechanism, the harmonics of vocal tones are being analyzed and presented to our con-sciousness as vowels. The intervals of the harmonic series must be deeply imbued in our unconscious. This is surely why people all round the world respond intuitively to the basic harmonic intervals, and why they are at the basis of every musical system. Some people, on first learning about the harmonic series and in hearing it played, feel an instant kinship with this hierarchy of pure intervals. It is, after all, our most direct perception of the numbers which underlie not just the acoustical world, but the whole physical universe.18*

Quite a large topic to contemplate! In essence, the vow-els offer an intimation of the archetypal expressions of the creative energies of the universe as they express themselves via the universal properties of acoustics. The gateway to this realm may be opened via something already at hand—you've already been using the vowels your entire life! Although we will next proceed to relating the vowels to the esoteric energy centers of the chakras, another advantage of the vowels is that

---

18. Joscelyn Godwin, *The Mystery of the Seven Vowels: In Theory and Practice* (Grand Rapids, MI: Phanes Press, 1991), 16.

they will have their power completely separate from any specific belief systems. Vowel sounds are found in every language on the planet. They are pure units of sonic energy, and they are therefore nondenominational and "safe" to work with. Regardless of any beliefs by any of the various sacred traditions on the planet, they are impossible to link with any one tradition. They will not clash with anyone's particular beliefs. The vowels are universal sounds, and they can therefore be used to teach bodily resonance and even resonance of the energy centers without going into potentially "foreign" terminology that may not be acceptable in certain belief systems.

Frequency Plus Intent

In his early researches in the field of sound healing, Jonathan Goldman exhaustively studied all available systems of toning to vibrate and resonate the chakras. He presented several of the most noteworthy ones in his book *Healing Sounds*, which includes systems by other pioneers in the sound field such as Randall McClellan, Kay Gardner, and Peter Michael Hamel. However, over the course of his studies, Goldman was struck by the wide variety of tones used to resonate chakras. The contemplation of different systems yielded many discrepancies and contradictions. This observation initially resulted in a state of confusion, but ultimately it led to a fundamental realization that helped coin his seminal formula "Frequency plus Intent = Healing."

The outlook prescribes that it is not the sound alone that creates a certain effect, but the sound in combination with the intent, or the focus of a practitioner's consciousness, which determines the outcome of an intonation. Keep this perspective in mind as you perform the exercise below. The focus of your attention and awareness on each chakra center will work in synergy with the sound you create.

It is still crucial to honor the importance of the sound! The formula is not merely "Intent = Healing." The physical resonance of the sound is also significant. One of the advantages of using sound as a form of energy work is that it is a physical plane force. Sound literally shakes and moves cells and molecules. Hence, the power of sound is a tool to influence subtle energy centers. Sound and intent form a powerful holistic synergy that is greater in effect than either one separately.

Chakra Mantras

As a result of his research, Jonathan Goldman created an original synthesis of the various systems of chakra toning. His approach involved assigning a specific vowel sound to each of the seven chakras. As he freely admits in *Healing Sounds*, it is only one possible system, but it contains a number of virtues that make it one of the more appealing systems of sonic chakra resonance.

One of the strengths of this system is that it follows a rising scale of harmonics. As noted in the quote from Joscelyn Godwin above, the vowel sounds naturally trigger specific harmonics. As you open your ears to hear them, you will discover that each vowel has subtle additional frequencies within the tone that stems off their fundamental pitch. These are the natural harmonics triggered by each unique vowel sound. The chosen vowel sequence naturally taps into an ascending harmonic series that contributes to its energetic patterning resonance.

In his years of acting as the advisor for Jonathan Goldman's Healing Sounds Correspondence Course, Alec has done personal one-on-one consultations with hundreds of participants who have experienced this exercise. If the measure of any sound experience lies in its value to provide positive personal results, then this system stands on a solid foundation. It is always an honor to share in the extraordinary results that can be triggered by this set of tones. We will now share it so that you can experience its resonance in the laboratory of your own being.

In the following exercise, the vowel sounds will be toned on a series of rising pitches starting with the lowest pitch you can sound and ending at the very highest pitch that you can sustain. Note that toning at the extreme high and low of your vocal register may be challenging at first, but above all, keep in mind that the most important guideline is to never force or strain your voice. If you initially have difficulty on the high or low end, simply allow the tones to ride gently on the breath, almost like lightly articulated exhalations.

Do not be concerned about the volume of your outward projection or worry if you're going high or low enough. The sounds you naturally make will be your own resonant frequencies, and the focus of your intent will also enhance the effect of the sound. As you become more familiar with the exercise, you will likely find that you will be able to relax your voice into a higher or lower register. But for this first time, simply make sure you are creating gentle and comfortable sounds.

The chakra toning exercise below uses the following sounds. Before you begin, take a few moments to familiarize yourself with the pronunciations.

The vowel sound for the root chakra is *uh*
  (as in the word *cup*).

The vowel sound for the second chakra is *ooo*
  (as in the word *you*).

The vowel sound for the navel chakra is *oh*
  (as in the word *go*).

The vowel sound for the heart chakra is *ah*
  (as in the word *father*).

The vowel sound for the throat chakra is *eye*
  (as in the word *my*).

The vowel sound for the third eye chakra is *aye*
  (as in the word *may*).

The vowel sound for the crown chakra is *eee*
  (as in the word *me*).

Exercise: Chakra Toning

Your complete attention is necessary for this exercise, so find a safe space where you can make sounds undisturbed for the duration of the session. Set a space where you will be able to experience deep meditation. Find a comfortable position, sitting either on the floor or in a chair. Be aware of your posture and keep your spine as straight as possible. You may put your hands in any position that is comfortable—on your knees or in your lap, or you may put them over the part of your body where you are resonating the sound. This placement serves to amplify the effects of the sounding and helps focus intention.

When you tone, use one complete breath with each vowel. You will tone each of the sacred vowel sounds seven times for each chakra and then be in silence at the end of this exercise.

To begin, focus your attention on the root chakra, located at the base of your spine. The vowel sound for this chakra is an *uh* sound. Imagine that you are breathing energy into this center to further target your awareness on this chakra. To find your starting pitch, first begin with a quiet hum. Let the tone of your hum drop to the lowest pitch you can comfortably sustain. When you've got it locked in, open your mouth and let your hum transform into the open voiced vowel.

If you would like to add color visualization to this sound, use the color red. Close your eyes while making the sound and focus your intention so that you visualize the sound resonating at the base of your spine. Feel the sound vibrating that area of your body and in your first chakra. Become aware that this chakra is being activated, balanced, and aligned with sacred sound.

Now tone the *uh* seven times. After you are finished, continue to breathe in and out of your root chakra. Feel for a subtle silent echo of the sound continuing to resonate this center.

Next focus your attention on the second chakra, located about three inches below your navel. Begin breathing energy in and out of this area. The vowel sound for this chakra is an *ooo* sound. To find your pitch, first return to humming the note you used for the root chakra. Let the pitch of your hum drift slowly upward until you feel an intuitive "click" that you are now sounding the appropriate pitch for the second chakra. Don't overthink it! Just be in the sound and feel. Know that the pitch you end up on will be the appropriate tone to resonate this chakra at this point in time.

A color that will complement the visualization for this sound is orange. Close your eyes while making the sound and focus your intention so that you visualize the sound resonating in the area about three inches below your navel and in your second chakra. Become aware that this chakra is being balanced and aligned and harmonized with the first chakra through toning the sacred vowel sounds.

Tone the *ooo* seven times. Repeat the brief pause for silent meditation when you are finished.

Now focus your attention on the navel chakra, located at the navel area and several inches above. Begin breathing energy in and out of this area. Repeat the rising hum technique to find your pitch, but this time begin on the note you used for the second chakra and let your pitch drift upward until you feel you are on the appropriate tone for the solar plexus area. The vowel sound for this chakra is an *oh* sound. Yellow will complement your color visualization. Close your eyes while making this sound and focus your intention so that you visualize the sound resonating in your navel area and in your navel chakra. Become aware that this chakra is being balanced and aligned with the first and second chakras through toning the sacred vowel sounds.

Tone *oh* seven times. Meditate in silence for a few minutes while maintaining focus on the navel chakra.

Now focus your attention on the heart chakra, located in the middle of your chest, to the right of your physical heart. Begin breathing energy in and out of this area and repeat the rising hum technique to find your pitch, this time bridging between the solar plexus and the heart area. The vowel sound for this chakra is an *ah* sound. If you wish to add a color to complement this sound, use green. Close your eyes while making this sound, and focus your intention so that you visualize the sound resonating in the area of your chest and in your heart chakra. Become aware that this chakra is being balanced and aligned with the other chakras we've been resonating, through toning the sacred vowel sounds.

Tone *ah* seven times. Meditate in silence for a few minutes while maintaining focus on the heart chakra.

Now focus your attention on the throat chakra, located at the throat. Begin breathing energy in and out of this area. Repeat the rising hum technique to find your pitch. The vowel sound for this chakra is an *eye* sound. A color to complement this sound is sky blue. Close your eyes while making this sound, and focus your intention so that you visualize this sound resonating in your throat and your throat chakra. Become aware that this chakra is being balanced and aligned with the other chakras we have been resonating through toning the sacred vowel sounds.

Tone *eye* seven times. Meditate in silence for a few minutes while maintaining focus on the throat chakra.

Now focus your attention on the third eye, or brow chakra, located in your forehead between your eyes and slightly above them. Begin breathing energy in and out of this area. Repeat the rising hum technique to find your pitch. The vowel sound for this chakra is an *aye* sound. A color that works well with this sound is indigo. Close your eyes while making this sound, and focus your intention so that you visualize the sound resonating in the area of your forehead and in your third eye. Become aware that this chakra is being balanced and aligned with the other chakras we have been resonating, through toning the sacred vowel sounds.

Tone *aye* seven times. Then meditate in silence for a few minutes while maintaining focus on the third eye chakra.

Now focus your attention on the crown chakra, located at the top of your head. Begin breathing energy in and out of this area. Again hum upward until you hit the highest pitch that you can comfortably sustain. The vowel sound for the crown chakra is an *eee* sound. A color that is used here is purple. Close your eyes while making this sound, and focus your intention so that you visualize the sound resonating at the top of your head and in your crown chakra. Become aware that this chakra is being balanced and aligned and that all of your chakras are now balanced and aligned with each other through toning the sacred vowel sounds.

Tone *eee* seven times. Let your attention remain in this center while performing the final meditation below.

At the completion of this exercise, which should take approximately twenty minutes to experience, you may feel very lightheaded. You have been moving energy up the body and the etheric centers, from the root to the crown chakra. With your chakras aligned and balanced, you might want to spend a longer period in deep meditation. After completing this exercise in group settings, we typically tell participants to take this opportunity to sit in silence and have the experience that will be for their highest benefit at this point in their spiritual development. This state can be a very nice place to be. Sit in a state of meditation and enjoy this experience. Allow yourself a good five to ten minutes for meditation. Enjoy!

When you are ready after completing your meditation, spend a few more minutes grounding yourself. In order to bring the energy back down into your body, first bring your attention back to the heart center area. Intone three midrange *ah* sounds, bringing the energy first down to your heart. Then tone three very deep *uh* sounds, bringing the energy down to your root chakra. Toning these sounds will immediately bring the energy back down into your physical body and help ground you.

Abbreviated Chakra Toning Exercises

Chakra toning is a wonderful exercise. We highly recommend creating the time to do the full experience. It would also be ideal to try it at different times of the day and note how your experience may vary. You may also find that the pitches you choose will be different depending on your state or energy level going into the exercise.

As noted with the five elements tonings, a few repetitions of the full-length meditation will serve to program the resonances into your being. You can then later access a similar balanced state much more quickly. If you would like to utilize chakra toning for a quick energy tune-up in the midst of your day, try the following variations:

- Do a shortened version of the chakra toning exercise by performing only one repetition of each vowel sound.

- Try doing this abbreviated version in the same sort of pitch-shifting fashion as the full-length exercise, or try it on one pitch, as was recommended with the bija mantras. In this variation, the rising harmonics within the vowels will serve to modulate areas of energetic resonance in lieu of shifting your fundamental pitch. Note any differences in your experience. Some people prefer the single pitch approach.

- Perform the toning sequence in one single breath. A slight bit of practice may be necessary in order to get the feel for pacing yourself so that you articulate all of the vowels evenly in a single breath, but you will quickly get the hang of it. Try the single breath chakra toning with a rising set of pitches that you feel intuitively as you ascend or perhaps focus on the steps of a major scale (i.e., the Do-Re-Mi-Fa-So-La-Ti-Do scale). Also try this approach on one single pitch.

Above all, have fun with these quick chakra toning variations! As you continue to work with the vowels, you may well be inspired to create new exercises of your own. In our modern society it's often difficult to create the space of fifteen minutes or half an hour to sound as a daily practice. These brief, but powerful, exercises can be a good alternative to doing no sound at all. As with many other types of energy work practices, these short sound experiences will have great cumulative effects if incorporated into your daily life with regularity rather than as sporadic isolated endeavors. They can be powerful tools for self-healing and transformation—particularly if you practice them daily.

Chakra Resonance via the Bija Mantras

As noted, the chakra toning exercise is a particularly powerful system of chakra resonance, but it is only one of many possibilities. Another potent sequence of tones to resonate the chakras is the bija mantras that were introduced in the last chapter. Indeed, the bija mantras are most commonly taught as a chakra toning system.

We find it useful to introduce the bijas as a more expansive system of working with archetypal energies, not limited to chakra center associations, yet it's important to call attention to this application of the bijas. The bija mantras are some of the most venerable and potent systems of chakra balancing. We invite you to experiment with them. Compare and contrast your experience with the bijas with the vowels as mantras. Neither system is better or worse; they are simply different approaches. We like them both, and we utilize them both at different times depending on the setting.

Chakra Chanting with the Bija Mantras

Some slight tweaks are needed in order to expand the five bija system to account for all of the chakras. The classic bija system typically does not include sounds for the third eye and crown. We like the following popular system:

Root Chakra: Tone the bija Lam

Sacral Chakra: Tone the bija Vam

Solar Plexus Chakra: Tone the bija Ram

Heart Chakra: Tone the bija Yam

Throat Chakra: Tone the bija Ham

Third Eye Chakra: Tone the syllable Sham

Crown Chakra: Tone the syllable Aum

To use the bija as chakra resonators, basically follow the instructions for the Chakra Toning exercise but substitute the appropriate bija for each chakra center instead of the recommended vowels. The bijas seem to feel more powerful when performed all on one pitch. Feel free to find a tone that works best for you. A pitch in the midrange of your vocal register typically yields the best results, but feel free to try low and high tones as well. Just stay on the same pitch throughout the whole bija sequence.

We recommend starting with this approach, but feel free to try the pitch-shifting method, if you would like. You may also wish to review the five elements bija toning exercises that were presented in the last chapter. Use your own creativity to incorporate elements of those meditations into your experience with the intention of drawing the appropriate elemental energies into each chakra for your highest benefit.

An Additional Note on Energy Circulation

As we have already noted, there are many concepts and models for subtle energy flow throughout the body. The vertical chakra system that we have worked with so far is only one of them. This system is an excellent model of mind/body psychology, but when doing practical work with energy centers in the body, it is always crucial to remember to harmoniously circulate any energies that may become activated. We have seen countless cases of people working with sonic energies and reporting head rushes or a feeling of floating. This is usually due to the person bringing a continually growing amount of energy upward. If this energy is not recirculated, the energy can build up and create imbalances. This extremely common issue is easily aided with the simple knowledge of techniques to allow this energy to flow in a continuous cycle through the body. One ideal system for this is known as the Microcosmic Orbit.

The Microcosmic Orbit derives from Taoist energy work teachings. The full complexity of the system is beyond the scope of this chapter. For more information, we would refer you to Mantak Chia's book *Awaken Healing Energy Through the Tao*. In a nutshell, the Microcosmic Orbit describes a circuit of energy that begins in the area of the root chakra and proceeds to flow upward along the back of the body. Upon reaching the crown, the circuit shifts to flowing downward along a channel in the front part of the body. There is a crucial switch in the area of the palate that makes the connection between the front and back channels. Touching the tip of your tongue to the area slightly behind your front teeth completes the circuit, creating a harmonious flow of energy that flows downward, eventually reconnecting with the source point at the root. The orbit continues to flow in a harmoniously circulating fashion, up and down, and back again.

But one need not know all of the details of the Microcosmic Orbit in order to experience energy circulation benefits. One way is to simply perform the vocal siren. If you wish to refresh your memory about the basics of this technique, please refer back to the introduction to the vocal siren in chapter 6. Sirening can be a powerful vocal warm-up method, but with a little added intention and attention, it can also be a very powerful toning technique for energy circulation. While you do the toning, imagine that there is a current of energy flowing up the back of your body as you ascend in pitch, and then back downward as you descend.

This technique is very useful to assist with the balancing of any energies that may be aroused during any type of sound or energy work practices. Such workings can often result in various types of physical sensations that may sometimes be indications of areas where energy may be stuck or not flowing in an ideal fashion. For example, if one ever feels lightheaded or "spacy" at any point during a practice, it is often a sign that too much energy has accumulated in the head (crown chakra) area. A few quick rounds of the Microcosmic Orbit technique are a simple but powerful method for integrating energy in a harmoniously balanced way.

The siren can be done on any sound, but a good one to experiment with first is the *ah* tone. Begin with the lowest *ah* that you can comfortably hit, and siren upward in a long full breath until you reach your highest pitch. Then siren downward until you reach your lowest comfortable tone. All the while, imagine the energy flowing up the back of your body on the ascending pitch and down the front on the descending tone. If it is comfortable for you to do so, add the piece of touching your tongue to that point slightly behind your front teeth. With a little practice, you should be able to easily sustain the *ah* sound with your tongue in this position. The importance of completing the two circuits with this tongue "lock" is stressed in the Taoist tradition. Try the siren both with and without the tongue position, and note if you feel any difference.

After you have practiced this method for a bit and have begun to feel the sensation of the up and down energy flows, try the variation of doing the ascending and descending siren all in one breath.

As yet another possibility, instead of an open voiced sound such as *ah,* do the Microcosmic Orbit sirening using a closed mouth humming sound. Try a gentle *mmm* tone, following the same approaches described above. Note any differences in your experience. For some people, this quieter, more internally directed sound enhances the subtle energy sensations.

Final Thoughts

Have fun with these chakra exercises! As we've noted a number of times, we encourage you to actually go back and perform the tonings. The main teachings will come via being in the sound current, not from the words on these pages. And, as always, the best results come from doing the sounding with a relaxed, playful, exploratory spirit.

We suggest first trying all the exercises we've recommended. But then feel free to experiment with your own variations as you feel inspired to do so. For example, you may wish to work with resonating each chakra separately by spending a whole session focusing on one center. If you follow this approach, we would recommend ending the session with a bit of Microcosmic Orbit sirening in order to circulate any energy that may become aroused harmoniously throughout your entire field.

The possibilities are endless! Know that as you balance and align your chakras with sacred sound, you are tuning your entire human instrument. Think of it as intonating the notes in your own personal scale of being. As you do so, you are honing and refining the vibrations that you project out into the world.

Recommended Reading

Awaken Healing Energy through the Tao: The Taoist Secret of Circulating Internal Power by Mantak Chia

A Chakra & Kundalini Workbook: Psycho-Spiritual Techniques for Health Rejuvenation, Psychic Powers, and Spiritual Realization by Jonn Mumford

Chakra Frequencies: Tantra of Sound by Jonathan and Andi Goldman

Wheels of Life: A User's Guide to the Chakra System by Anodea Judith

Wheels of Light by Rosalyn Bruyere

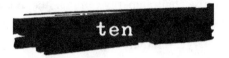

ten

The Sound of Magick

It's All In Your Head...
You just have no idea how big your head is!
—LON MILO DUQUETTE

N ow that we have touched on a few methods for using
sound to activate energy and harmonize various energetic centers, let's move on to consider other ways sound can
be used to facilitate shift and change. We have already noted
how everything is in a state of vibration and all phenomena
can be thought of as operating within various bandwidths of
energetic frequencies. Therefore a key metaphor for facilitating change could be to think in terms of "frequency shifting." We owe this concept to the idea expressed in the title of
the Jonathan Goldman book *Shifting Frequencies.*

The most expansive lesson of working with sound may
be that we are all unique vibratory beings who are fluid in
nature. As a result, we are subject to great potential for shift

and change in frequency. Recall the points we raised in the discussion of the chakra energy centers. Just as chakras are not static objects or things, we are also ultimately just vibrating fields of energy. Yes, there is a certain physical reality that would be foolish to deny, but the study of energy medicine reveals that this physical bandwidth is only one aspect of our being. There are also complex, multidimensional subtle fields to consider that interrelate and influence each other in an intricate symphony of vibration. Indeed, as is seriously proposed in the outlooks of quantum mechanics, these fields may represent higher orders of reality that exert potent influence on the observable physical plane. The revelation that the universe is not an assembly of physical parts but instead comes from an entanglement of immaterial energy waves stems from the work of Albert Einstein, Max Planck, and Werner Heisenberg, amongst others.

To take things a step further, one's consciousness plays a profound role in the way these energies are shaped and experienced. This claim is not mere speculation—quantum physicists have discovered that physical atoms are made up of vortices of energy that are constantly spinning and vibrating. Matter, at its tiniest currently observable level, is energy, and human consciousness is connected to it. Human consciousness can influence its behavior and even restructure it. A quote attributed to the seminal quantum theorist Niels Bohr sums up all of the above with the line, "Everything we call real is made of things that cannot be regarded as real."[19]

---

19. Arjun Walla, "The Illusion of Matter: Our Physical Material World Isn't Really Physical at All." Collective Evolution, accessed December 5, 2013. http://tinyurl.com/kfcvykb.

So what is real? Perhaps consciousness itself is the source of the ultimate reality? This speculation echoes the cosmological roots of the Samkhya philosophy we discussed in the five elements chapter. Another concise statement of this outlook is offered by the author R. C. Henry:

> A fundamental conclusion of the new physics also acknowledges that the observer creates the reality. As observers, we are personally involved with the creation of our own reality. Physicists are being forced to admit that the universe is a "mental" construction. Pioneering physicist Sir James Jeans wrote: "The stream of knowledge is heading toward a non-mechanical reality; the universe begins to look more like a great thought than like a great machine. Mind no longer appears to be an accidental intruder into the realm of matter, we ought rather hail it as the creator and governor of the realm of matter. Get over it, and accept the inarguable conclusion. The universe is immaterial—mental and spiritual.[20]

All of the above claims bring us to a fascinating crossroads. The field of energy medicine basically consists of techniques by which the focus of consciousness can shape energy and thus influence matter. This is the essence of frequency shifting! For just as one can turn the dial on a radio to receive a complete new bandwidth of frequencies, the modulation of our own physical, emotional, and psychological frequencies can yield a wealth of benefits.

---

20. R. C. Henry, "The Mental Universe." NATURE 436 (July 7, 2005): 29.

It's also exciting to realize that the claims of energy practitioners are being supported by the cutting edge of conventional science. As awareness of energy medicine continues to gain more popular acceptance, we will see more extraordinary practical applications of these quantum theories for health and wellness. Contemplation of the energy field truly presents a groundbreaking fusion of elements from cutting-edge science merged with the knowledge and techniques from ancient bodies of knowledge such as shamanism. Yet here is another vast wellspring of knowledge rooted in the Western esoteric tradition that is less commonly discussed. This is the field of magick.

What Is Magick?

Magick, spelled with a *k* to denote a distinction from the entertainment-oriented practices of stage magic, has been called the "Yoga of the West." Similar to yoga, magick offers a profound array of practices and techniques for both personal enhancement as well as spiritual evolution and attainment. The study of magick offers great rewards for energy practitioners. In fact, many contemporary systems of energy work and mind/body/spirit self-development owe a great debt to the magickal traditions, but rarely honor this source.

We have referred to the importance of intention a number of times. It's one thing to state the importance of focusing intent in order to achieve results with energy medicine. But that claim begs the question—how does one focus intent? Familiarity with the fundamental concentration and visualization practices in the realm of magick can serve to provide such skill. The ability to achieve more finely tuned levels of focus can only serve to enhance one's abilities as a practitioner. While all positive energetic intentions definitely have positive value, think of the difference between the qualities of light from a low-watt bulb versus a finely tuned laser. Magick is a vast field of study drawing from many centuries worth of sources and practices. Our goal here is simply to introduce you to some basic definitions and concepts.

Definitions of Magick

For our purposes here, let's establish a working concept of magick. The classic definition is: "Magick is the Science and Art of causing Change to occur in conformity with Will."[21] However, later practitioners felt compelled to elaborate on this definition. The celebrated occult author and psychologist Dion Fortune added an extra dimension saying, "Magick is the Science and Art of causing changes in consciousness to occur in conformity with Will."[22] This definition harmonizes with our theme. The only universe you will ever truly experience is the universe that is represented by your own consciousness. Therefore, if you are able to change your own consciousness, then the universe will change. Another one of the most profound (and sanest) contemporary writers on the subject of magick, Lon Milo DuQuette, states, "Personally, I've come to the realization that the only real changes I can

---

21. Aleister Crowley, *Magick: Liber ABA Book Four*, 2nd rev. ed., ed. Hymenaeus Beta (York Beach, ME: Weiser Books, 1997), 126.

22. Donald Michael Kraig, *Modern Magick: Twelve Lessons in the High Magickal Arts*, rev. ed. (Woodbury, MN: Llewellyn Publications, 2010), 14.

effect with magick are changes in myself. By changing myself, I change the world around me, hopefully for the better."²³

If the essence of magick is to skillfully modulate our consciousness, then sound offers a valuable bridge, for sound is a powerful tool both to generate energy and to alter our own consciousness. And as noted in the quote above, as we change ourselves, our perception of the world changes, and thus our experience in the world changes.

Sound and Magick

The field of magick contains a vast array of practices pertaining to the alteration and enhancement of consciousness, as well as techniques for such things as making contacts with various spiritual entities and journeying to other planes of existence. The use of sound in the form of chanting and specialized intonations plays a major role in many of these esoteric traditions. In fact, these associations are still hinted at in commonplace expressions. Think of the word *abracadabra*. These days it's just a comical conjuror's catchphrase with no force behind it, like *hocus pocus* and other meaningless utterances. But the word actually derives from an Aramaic phrase meaning "I will create as I speak." The phrase *abracadabra* is extremely ancient and originally was thought to be a powerful invocation with mystical powers. For one illustration of this theme, recall the opening chapters of the King James translation of the book of Genesis. One of the early verses contains

---

23. Lon Milo DuQuette, *Enochian Vision Magick: An Introduction and Practical Guide to the Magick of Dr. John Dee and Edward Kelley* (York Beach, ME: Weiser, 2008), xxviii.

the line "And God *said*, Let there be light: and there was light."
Here we have a metaphor for creation via the spoken word!

As we've noted previously, sound is universally hailed as a
creative force in many spiritual traditions. This concept can be
extended to the creative and transformative power of speech.
When a layperson thinks of magick, they may well think of
spells and enchantments. And, in a sense, this association is
correct. In fact, the word *enchant* stems from the Latin root
incantare, which means "to sing or chant magical words or
sounds."

However, we do not need to venture off into distant esoteric realms to experience the magickal power of speech. We
can encounter it in everyday language! In a significant sense,
all language is magick. Language is both an expression of our
consciousness and serves to shape how our consciousness perceives reality.

The school of psychology known as Neuro-Linguistic Pro-
gramming (NLP) delves deeply into this topic. For example,
think of the difference between the phrases "I hear what you're
saying," "I see what you mean," and "I grasp your point." They
all basically mean "I understand you," yet each one reveals
a different circuit of perception. We all perceive the world
through the basic sensory modalities of sight, sound, touch,
taste, and smell. NLP examines how the language we choose is
often a reflection of our preferred mode of perception. In the
example above, the person using the word "see" is expressing a
preference for the visual mode of perception, "hear" indicates a
dominance of the auditory sense, and "grasp" implies a leaning
toward perceiving the world in terms of bodily (or kinesthetic)
sensations.

Each of these terms expresses a different bandwidth of consciousness. So the first practical application of sonic magick could be to tune in to the language that people use. Take the time to really listen, both to the actual words and to the subtle energetics of other people's expressions. One way of gaining rapport, or coming into greater harmony, with another person is to take note of the type of sensory-based language they use to express themselves and use similar phrases yourself during your communications. In NLP, this preference is known as the Lead Representational System. This exercise in matching language patterns may serve as an important technique for harmoniously resonating with another person's state of consciousness.

Above and beyond the implications of word choices, everyday language also expresses aspects of energetic intention. Our thoughts are powerful. Our words conduct our thoughts. Every time we say something, we are transmitting energy with those words. But the literal words used are just the tip of the iceberg of the multidimensional levels of our interactions. Communication specialists have estimated that people only respond to 7 percent of the literal verbal content of communication. The source for this commonly quoted statistic is the work of Dr. Albert Mehrabian, the author of *Silent Messages*.

Dr. Mehrabian found that 7 percent of any message is conveyed through words, 38 percent through certain vocal elements, and 55 percent through nonverbal elements (facial expressions, gestures, posture, etc.).[24] We would also add

---

24. Albert Mehrabian, *Silent Messages: Implicit Communication of Emotions and Attitudes* (Belmont, CA: Wadsworth, 1971).

intuition to that list. To varying degrees, everyone is capable of sensing subtle energetics behind words, sometimes in contradiction to their literal meaning. For example, have you ever been in a social situation where you had to interact with someone with whom you had some history of conflict? The person may approach you and say something along the lines of "Lovely to see you!" yet you end up with a feeling of distaste and discomfort. Here is a case where the intention behind the words did not match the surface level statement.

This phenomenon illustrates another lesson in everyday sonic magick. It is important to be mindful that the intent behind our communication matches the literal meaning of our words. People will sense the difference! As Steven Halpern has written, "Sound is a carrier wave of consciousness." [25] There is always more information content attached to and broadcasted on the sound waves of words than their mere literal meaning.

Contemplation along these lines brings us into the sphere of a third refinement of the definition of magick. The occultist Donald Michael Kraig adds an important dimension saying, "Magick is the science and art of causing change (in consciousness) to occur in conformity with will, using means not currently understood by traditional Western science." [26] This added element implying the transmission of information or the causation of effects by seemingly "supernatural" means is what people most commonly associate with magick.

---

25. Steven Halpern, "Healing Vibrations," *Yoga Journal*, no. 114 (1994): 122.
26. Donald Michael Kraig, *Modern Magick*, 15.

Messages from Water

Can words transmit energy and cause effects in a fashion not currently understood by traditional Western science? Certain recent studies seem to indicate that they can. One noteworthy example is a series of experiments conducted in the 1990s by Masaru Emoto.[27]

The focus of Dr. Emoto's work was to document the effects of intention on the structure of water. The essence of his methodology consisted of taking samples of water from various sources and freezing individual droplets in order to observe the structure of the ice crystals formed. The droplets of water were frozen under special conditions that allowed them to be photographed. Dr. Emoto found that water from pure, fresh sources produced beautifully shaped hexagonal crystals, whereas water from polluted sources formed distorted disharmonious shapes.

At first, he observed crystals of tap water, river water, and lake water. From the city tap water he could not get any aesthetically pleasing crystals that were unique in design. Furthermore, the water from rivers or lakes that surrounded big cities also produced unpleasant shapes. But water from rivers and lakes far away from developed areas produced crystals that had vibrant uniqueness and beautiful symmetry.

These initial observations seemed to indicate that in addition to the effects of chemical pollution, the structure of water seemed to be influenced by the vibrations of its environment. But the next evolutions of Dr. Emoto's work took an even more extraordinary turn. He began to expose samples of pure,

---

27. Masaru Emoto, *The Hidden Messages in Water* (Hillsboro, OR: Beyond Words, 2004).

distilled water to different pieces of music. He was stunned to find that the crystals formed by water exposed to beautiful, harmonious music produced clear, finely structured crystals. In sharp contrast, water that was immersed in angry or harsh music produced distorted shapes similar to that of polluted water. The strong indication was that the energetics of the music had a direct effect on the structure of water.[28]

The implications of Dr. Emoto's discoveries are extremely thought provoking, especially when we consider the vast amount of Earth's surface that is covered by water and the fact that the human body consists of about 70 percent water. Water is vital to all life. The fact that the molecular structure of the water can be affected by our consciousness, our intent, and our sounds is extremely important and may have great implications for the future of personal and planetary harmony and healing.

One of Dr. Emoto's more ambitious experiments drives this point home even more strongly. In another phase of his work, very polluted and toxic water was taken from the area of the Fujiwara Dam in Japan. In the first rounds of testing, the water produced the expected unpleasantly distorted shapes. Dr. Emoto then had Buddhist monks pray and chant over the water. In the follow-up tests, the water formed the beautiful clear crystals similar to water from pristine sources. This series of experiments seems to demonstrate how chanting with focused intent appears to have the ability to transmute and purify water. It's an example of an incantation that causes change to occur in conformity with will.

---

28. Hado USA, "Water Crystals Gallery," http://hadousa.com /gallery.html.

But as astounding as this case study was, the next phase of Dr. Emoto's work was even more extraordinary. In the next phase of experiments, Dr. Emoto began to simply attach pieces of paper containing various words and phrases to the outside of vials of distilled water. He found results that paralleled his experiments with the effects of music. Incredibly enough, phrases such as "Love and Gratitude" and "Thank you" produced stunningly beautiful crystals. Harsh words such as "You fool" and "You disgust me" created harsh, sludgy shapes.

How is it that mere words on slips of paper seemed to affect the physical structure of water? It's certainly not because the water was able to read the messages! A possible explanation could be gleaned from the concept from the magickal traditions known as thought forms. A thought form is basically a construct of energy created by the consciousness of a practitioner that assumes a sort of independent existence. It's as if the vivid imagining of an idea or entity causes it to become real. To relate back to sound, the thought form could be conceived of as a certain waveform or pattern of energetic vibration. Once they are created, the energy of thought forms can be transferred via various methods. In the case of Dr. Emoto's work, the writing of the words seems to transfer the vibration of the thought form behind them directly to the physical substance of the water. Simply writing the word *love* seemed to convey the positive energy of the emotion to the water crystals, which had beneficial results on their energetic patterning and ultimately their physical structure.

Sonic Affirmations

To bring the relevance of these thoughts even closer to home, note that a large percentage of our body mass also consists of water. Dr. Emoto's work seems to demonstrate powerful dimensions of our thought and intentions. The power of this realization indicates both great responsibility and awesome possibility. If the simple writing of basic phrases on slips of paper can alter physical structure, how can we apply these principles to benefit our own lives?

In recent years, there has been a lot of information released into public awareness pertaining to the Law of Attraction and various manifestation techniques. The book and movie *The Secret* were a couple of the most popular and influential works in this realm. The Law of Attraction is basically a simplified magickal technique that can be understood in terms of sound. The fundamental principle is that if you can tune your thoughts, beliefs, and energy patterns in alignment with a certain desire or outcome, then that desire or outcome will manifest in your life. In essence, it's a subtler manifestation of the principles of resonance and entrainment. If you can resonate the vibration of a particular desire, then the universe will begin to entrain to that frequency and bring it into being in the realm of your experience.

But the ideas expressed in works such as *The Secret* are not new. Many of them can be traced back to early works in the self-help field such as *Think and Grow Rich* by Napoleon Hill and *The Master Key System* by Charles Haanel as well as the distillation of Western esoteric philosophy found in *The Kybalion* by the Three Initiates. Indeed, the classic aphorism

"thoughts are things" coined by Napoleon Hill strongly resonates with the ideas we have been discussing. Thoughts are
not ephemeral wisps in the mind, but have a palpable reality
that is directly capable of influencing our physical world and
being.

Affirmations

A common technique found in the Law of Attraction involves
the use of affirmations. Affirmations can be thought of as
magickal phrases. They are statements of intent crafted to
cause change in accordance with your will. A simple example
is a statement such as "I can do it," which is an acknowledg-
ment of the synergy between thought and sound. Yet, unfortunately, a common criticism of the practice of affirmations
is that they don't work! Many people never experience the
results they are trying to affirm in a satisfactory way. How can
one improve these results? Like so many things, the key lies in
simplicity.

The simpler the intent, the easier it is to focus and manifest. Complex intents often contain contradictions and distractions. The problem is that many statements fail to pass
beyond the conscious mind level. It has been said that 90
percent of our brain capabilities are subconscious while only
10 percent is conscious. In relation to our current topic, the
only real ability of our conscious mind is the power to act
as a sort of lens to focus attention and intention. The truly
awesome powers of our consciousness lie in the much vaster
unconscious mind.

In order to penetrate and activate the powers of the
unconscious mind, one must direct energy and intent to it in
an efficient fashion. Verbal phrases are rarely completely suf-

ficient. The subconscious mind is more susceptible to vivid imagination and strong emotion. We will elaborate on these methods shortly, but first we must consider how to create a proper space for such workings.

Sonic Space Clearing

A major facet of practice in the various magickal traditions involves the use of ritual. Ritual basically involves the establishment of a space and setting in which to perform various activities intended to cultivate or attract desired energies. In a sense, ritual could be thought of as the construction of a radio receiver in order to receive or broadcast certain desired frequencies.

The most basic ritual practice involves a banishing ritual, the purpose of which is to clear the space you are operating in of any unwanted energies and, in turn, to charge the space with positive beneficial energies that will support your intention. Banishing is closely related to the energy medicine practice of "space clearing," which is usually intended to accomplish similar ends.

On a side note, one simple method for space clearing via sound is to use sharp percussive sounds. Such sounds can serve to break up energy fields and patterns. The use of rattles or bells or simply clapping your hands can be very effective for this end.

In the magick traditions, banishing rituals can range from a simple imagining of white light permeating a space to more elaborate operations such the Lesser Banishing Ritual of the Pentagram, which involves more intricate visualizations and the intonation of specific divine names. Here we will offer a simple toning ritual that will serve this purpose.

The foundation of our ritual will be the emotions of love and gratitude. We have seen the positive effects of that phrase on the structure of water in Dr. Emoto's work. A common technique for manifestation involves the visualization of one's desire as if it has already happened while offering gratitude for it along with the affirmation that it has already come to pass. We will use these thought forms in combination.

In the following ritual, we will focus on the heart center and use the tone *ah*. There are several reasons for this choice. First of all, interesting research conducted by the Heart Math Institute has shown that the heart broadcasts the most potent electromagnetic field, a field that operates at a massively stronger amplitude than that of the brain. In addition, certain focused breathing techniques such as the one below can serve to create an increased coherence between the electromagnetic fields of the heart and brain, which result in enhanced states of balance and well-being.

The *ah* tone is a perfect choice to complement this heart focus. First of all, the *ah* sound is one of the easiest tones for people to create. It is almost universally regarded in different traditions as a heart sound—a sound for resonating the heart center and embodying compassion and love. It is also simply a primary vowel sound and thus, while being quite sacred, it can be utilized by any tradition, regardless of beliefs or language. The *ah* is thus unconsciously understood to be a sound without borders; it can be utilized by anyone, regardless of race, creed, tradition, or religion without people having prior concepts of what it means. For most, there is an unconscious positive feeling during the sound that naturally resonates in and from the heart. It is a sound we frequently make when we're in love or when we're feeling a deep sense of peace.

In addition to these natural associations, the *ah* sound is a sacred seed syllable. It is found in many of the god and goddess names on the planet (Tara, Buddha, Krishna, Yahweh, Allah), as well as many of the sacred words (Amen, alleluia, Aum). Most mystical traditions worldwide also find it to be the sound of the heart chakra. Yet in spite of these connections to spiritual traditions, since *ah* is simply a pure vowel sound, it defies denomination or description as a mantra and is acceptable by everyone. If you take nothing else away from this chapter, we hope that you will still always recall the *ah* tone is perhaps one of the most powerful universal intonations for energy enhancement.

Exercise: The *Ah* Ritual

To begin, find yourself in a space where you will not be disturbed. Assume a comfortable position with your spine erect. This could be a meditation posture or simply seated in a straight-backed chair. When you are ready, bring your attention to your heart area in the center of your chest. While maintaining this focus, begin breathing energy into your heart area. On the in breath, imagine that a current of energy is flowing into your heart. On the out breath, feel a current of energy flowing out from your heart. This is the Heart Math technique that begins to establish the enhanced state of heart/brain coherence.

After a few moments, begin to tone the *ah* sound. Use a gentle, flowing tone of voice on a comfortable note in the easy midrange of your vocal register. Tone the *ah* sound for several moments while continuing to feel the energetic flow in and out of your heart area.

As you sound, begin to think of something in your life for which you feel gratitude and appreciation. It could be a loved one, a beloved pet, a cherished possession, or a past accomplishment. It could simply be a basic daily experience such as a beautiful sunrise or a pleasant excursion in nature. There are many possibilities. Simply tune in to something that evokes a deep sense of gratitude and appreciation for you. Concentrate on deeply sensing that feeling, and feel it permeate all the pores of your being.

When you feel that you have got a hold on this feeling, begin to imagine a golden sphere of energy expanding out from your heart. If you wish, you can instead imagine a sphere of pure white light. See and feel it growing in size until it expands out several feet from your body in all directions. See the sphere expand to dimensions slightly wider than your outstretched arms in a perfect sphere that encompasses your whole body with your heart at the center. As you continue to visualize the sphere and tone *ah*, imagine that the energy of the feeling of gratitude is also permeating outward from your heart to fill this space.

If your intention is simply to balance yourself, then let the sphere remain as it is. If you wish to clear the space you are in, proceed to imagine that the boundaries of the sphere continue to expand outward to fill the shape of the entire room. See and feel the energy of your visualization, sound, and gratitude filling the whole space, from wall to wall and from ceiling to floor.

After a few more moments in this state, let your voice fade to silence. Feel the new energy of the space, knowing that you have cleared, balanced, and aligned yourself and your surroundings with the energy of the *ah* tone.

A Final Definition of Magick

Without analyzing what happened during the exercise above too much, we'd like to present yet another definition of magick from Isaac Bonewits:

> *Magic is a science and an art comprising a system of concepts and methods for the build-up of human emotion, altering the electrochemical balance of the metabolism, using associational techniques and devices to concentrate and focus this emotional energy, thus modulating the energy broadcast by the human body.29*

This new spin on the definition of magick brings some new factors into account. The energy of emotion may be one

---

29. Philip Emmons Isaac Bonewits, *Real Magic: An Introductory Treatise on the Basic Principles of Yellow Magic*, rev. ed. (York Beach, ME: Weiser, 1989), 204.

of the most powerful driving forces for manifestation, for the subconscious responds very powerfully to emotional content. This energy can serve as a potent fuel to add more power to the practice of affirmations. Furthermore, this buildup of emotional charges can serve to shift the biochemistry of the body. This shift in turn alters one's electromagnetic field. As your personal energy field shifts, the energy you are capable of broadcasting also becomes more potent, particularly when working with the vibrations of love and appreciation as a starting point. This phenomenon offers major benefits both for affirmation practice and energy healing work in general.

Exercise: Energized Affirmations

To bring this concept into practical working, let's recall the basics of Dr. Emoto's work. In his experiments, the writing of a simple word or phrase was sufficient to cause physical change in the structure of water. Distilling an affirmation down to its simplest essence can serve to enhance its potency as a message to the unconscious mind. We will combine this concept with the evocation of feeling that we experienced in the *ah* toning exercise above.

To begin, think of something you would like to affirm. Distill the desire down to a simple phrase. One to three words would be ideal, but there are no limitations. Just note that this technique will work best with an affirmation of a single-digit number of words. Your affirmation could be for a quality you would like to manifest or embody such as "confidence" or "clear communication." It could also be for a condition you would like to attract such as "new job" or "loving relationship." There are many possibilities.

After you have decided on your aim and distilled it to a simple phrase, take a few minutes to imagine what it would feel like if your desire was already true. Don't merely think about it on a mental plane level. Truly feel it in your body. Imagine the sensations of energy flow you would feel in your body if your affirmation was already true. Feel that it is true and has already happened.

For the next step, perform the *ah* ritual described above. After you have completed, charged, and expanded your sphere, go into silence. Then begin to think about your affirmation phrase. Feel those sensations in your body as if your affirmation has already manifested and offer thanks. After you have tuned in to that feeling, begin to softly chant your affirmation in a gentle, flowing tone. Hear and feel the simple music of the words before the literal meaning. You may even find your affirmation morphing into a simple melody or song. Indeed, adding this component of pure sound can also facilitate broadcasting your intent to the unconscious. Sing your affirmations! Also recall that sound is a physical plane energy form. Vocalizing an affirmation provides it with an extra bridge to manifestation in the physical realm.

After a few moments of this practice, begin to feel the energy of your affirmation centering on and merging with your heart field. Feel your affirmation merging and harmonizing with your heart center. Feel your affirmed intention becoming enhanced and magnified by the coherent heart energy generated by the *ah* ritual. As you do so, recall those sensations of energy flow that you evoked when picturing that your affirmation has already come to pass. Feel those sensations begin to intensify and become enhanced with the gratitude evoked by the *ah* toning.

When you are ready, feel the energy of your affirmation expanding outward to fill your sphere. As you do so, know that the power of the waveform of your affirmation is continuing to be enhanced by the power of gratitude and is now being broadcast out to the universe. Continue flowing with this sensation and let your sphere expand. Let it fill the space where you currently find yourself, and then let it expand beyond. Let your sphere expand to the point where it feels like a bubble of energy surrounding the entire planet, and then beyond. Feel that the energy of your affirmation is like a pebble that has been thrown into a pond. Feel the ripples extend out in all directions and dimensions, eventually touching the farthest reaches of the universe.

Continue to enjoy this expanded state for as long as it feels appropriate as you continue intoning your affirmation. When you are ready, summon your sphere back. Imagine it shrinking back down to surround the planet, then return to your current space, and then back to its original dimensions. From there, let your sphere continue to contract until it surrounds your body like a second skin. And then let the energy of your sphere, along with all of the encoded energy of your affirmation, contract until it feels like a condensed crystal globe surrounding your heart.

After this final sensation clicks into place, let your chant fade to silence. Enjoy a quiet meditation for a few moments while continuing to let the feeling of gratitude resonate throughout all the levels of your being. When you feel complete, state out loud, "And so it is! I give thanks!" Then get up as quickly as you are able and move your body. Stretch your neck and shoulders. Begin to move. Make circles with your arms, shoulders, and hips. Stomp your feet and make some grounding sounds. Then move out of the space where you conducted your meditation. Perhaps step outside and get some fresh air and go for a short walk. While doing so, forget your affirmation—release it from your conscious mind.

The best follow-up to this working would be to now go enjoy some fun, distracting activity. But know that without requiring your conscious attention, your heart sphere is still broadcasting the waveform of your affirmation out to the universe. The first domino has been cast, which will cause your affirmation to resonate back into your reality.

Just as it is always important to honor the silence after the sound, it is important to close the doors of intention and put your goal out of your conscious mind once the working is complete. Focus your intention to perform the ritual and then put it aside in order to let some unconscious "cooking" take place.

If you think about your outcome too much afterward, you will run the risk of triggering conscious mind processes. This type of internal dialogue can serve to trigger overeager expectations and doubt, which can both function as types of negative affirmations that can run contrary to your goal.

Think of your ritual practice as planting an energetic seed. After you plant a seed, you must allow time for it to take root and grow naturally of its own accord. If you proceed to dig the seed up every day to double check if it's sprouting, you will ruin the process. Conscious-mind rumination about your ritual will likely spoil the process of manifestation. Plant your seeds and let them sprout! But do still feel free to occasionally sing to your flowers!

Recommended Reading

The Hidden Messages in Water by Masaru Emoto

The Kyballion by The Three Initiates

Modern Magick: Twelve Lessons in the High Magickal Arts by Donald Michael Kraig

Practical Sigil Magic: Creating Personal Symbols for Success by Frater U. D.

Real Magic: an Introductory Treatise on the Basic Principles of Yellow Magic by Isaac Bonewits

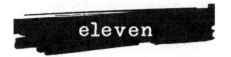

eleven

Words of Power:
The Magick of Mantra

We heal ourselves and we heal the planet,
we heal the planet and we heal ourselves.

—JONATHAN GOLDMAN

In the last chapter, we introduced some basic concepts from the Western esoteric tradition of magick. We would now like to consider another multifaceted discipline for shaping energy and consciousness—the practice of mantra. The art and science of mantra is a vast field of study ranging from simple, one-syllable tones to more elaborate phrases and intricate devotional songs. In fact, aspects of mantra practice relate back to the topic of the last chapter, for it's likely that the average layperson's primary association with magick would be the use of spoken spells chants, intonations, and "words of power." This connection is sound, for mantra can indeed be used for magickal purposes. And like magick, the applications of mantra are broad, ranging from spiritual development practices to practical personal manifestation.

However, this dual purpose may raise some questions as to whether or not using these techniques to manifest things for personal material benefits is appropriate. Indeed, such promise is what often initially attracts people to pursue various esoteric arts. In addition to its power for facilitating spiritual, intellectual, and psychological growth, mantra can also be used for such ends. But there is nothing inherently wrong with seeking personal benefits and rewards—as long as you take care to ensure that your intentions do not involve harm or taking advantage of others. Indeed, it may not be truly possible to do "higher," more "spiritual" work until one's material needs are adequately met. The pursuit of practical manifestation via the vehicle of mantra can offer beneficial safeguards, for mantras intoned with good-hearted positive intent can inherently attune all your practical work with the divine.

Definition of Mantra

The word *mantra* is a Sanskrit term derived from the roots *manas*, which means "to think," and *trai*, which means "to protect" or "to free from." *Mantra* can therefore mean "the thoughts that liberate and protect" or be thought of as a type of "mind protection." As a spiritual practice, mantra is intended to protect the mind from the distractions of worldly concerns and conceptions. And in this case, "mind" here refers to all six forms of consciousness—eye, ear, nose, tongue, body, and mental activity—which are ultimately all to be freed or protected from the mundane world in order to attain full enlightenment.

Mantras are sounds or words that when recited (either aloud or silently) have the ability to alter the consciousness of the reciter. In various spiritual traditions, the ultimate aim of the mantra is to unite the reciter with a particular deity or divine consciousness. While more commonly associated with various Eastern traditions, mantras are used by nearly every spiritual and religious path as a means of union with the sacred. Practically every path has some sort of exercise in which enlightenment may be achieved by chanting devotional names or phrases. Examples of phrases from the Christian tradition that could be utilized as mantras are Kyrie Elesison, Alleluia, Sanctus, and Agnus Dei. The Sufi tradition offers Hu, which can be viewed as an embodiment of the divine sound current of the cosmos.

As we noted in chapter 4, the usage of trance-inducing chants is prevalent in the shamanic traditions. But the most profound developments of mantra practice may be found in the Hindu/Vedic systems of Sanskrit mantra and the Tibetan Buddhist traditions. For our purposes, we would do well to examine the basics of this knowledge more thoroughly.

How Mantras Work

The basic premise behind the working of the mantra is very much the same principles we have discussed in earlier chapters—that of resonance and entrainment. Everything in the universe vibrates on specific wavelengths, including (at least conceptually) various psychic, spiritual, or divine entities.

Therefore a mantra could be thought of as a type of cosmic tuning fork. The repetition of a mantra allows the practitioner to attune his or her own resonance so that ultimately the use of the mantra will create an energetic entrainment with a particular deity or force.

Mantras could be thought of as sonic formulas. In a fashion similar to how chemical formulas can create particular elements through the addition of different substances, mantras can create a waveform of sonic energy that can serve to harmonize the consciousness of the practitioner with energy of the mantra. For example, in the case of a devotional mantra, the intonation can serve to trigger a resonance with the specific deity that allows one to come into union with its presence or qualities.

In the various source traditions, whether it be Vedic, Tibetan, or Hebrew, it is claimed that the use of mantras can cause union with divine beings, enlightenment, or attainment of fantastic powers and abilities (known as siddhis). The spiritual attributes and abilities that can be obtained or united with through mantra are potentially limitless.

This concept of morphogenetic fields of sound is a very real phenomenon that provides an explanation as to why chanting or listening to a mantra that has been intoned and resonated for thousands of years can be so powerful. The energy field created by such a sound continues to build and become more highly charged via continual sounding. This is one reason why it may be more difficult to work with mantras from ancient civilizations that are long gone. While the morphogenetic fields of the ancient sounds may still exist, they may need to be reactivated. It takes much more energy to activate and work with such sounds than to take advantage of an ongoing "alive" sound, as in the case of a mantra like the *om* that is continuously being activated and charged.

When Tibetan monks perform certain chants, they consciously work with their powers of visualization plus the energy of morphogenetic fields to empower thought forms of the divinities they seek to invoke. If one were to perform these same chants with the intention of opening to the possibility of traveling on the sound in this deepest level of chanting, it is quite possible to begin to resonate with these thought forms, whether or not you were previously consciously aware of their existence. They exist in some other realm of the collective unconscious or perhaps super-conscious. These higher levels of reality can be accessed through sound.

Some Sample Mantras

We will now offer some examples of mantras for you to work with so you can begin to have your own experience with this practice. We will first discuss the definitions, general usages, and pronunciations of each mantra. Afterward, we will offer some suggested approaches for you to begin to practice them.

Om (AUM)

Om is considered by many spiritual teachers and masters to be the original creative sound of the universe. The Vedic creator god Brahma is said to have uttered *om* when he created the many worlds and planes of existence. In this sense, *om* may have been the "word" that was uttered in a similar fashion to the Judeo-Christian concept of "In the Beginning was the Word." *Om* is often used as the single sound that will do the work and have the power of many other sounds due to its multidimensional resonances. *Om* is also found at the beginning of many longer mantric phrases as well as the beginning and end of most Sanskrit recitations, prayers, and texts. It is said that all other sounds can be found within the *om*.

This creative association is enhanced when *om* is pronounced in its three-syllable form. This three syllable *aum* is sometimes referred to as the tantric form of the mantra. In this approach the *O* is enunciated as a combination of *A* and *U*, so that *om* becomes a three-syllable world, as in *aah-oou-oohmm*. If the *aum* is pronounced slowly and mindfully, it actually makes a broad sweep through a full spectrum of harmonics. Notice how the mouth opens wide with the initial *A*, then gradually reduces as the *U* is pronounced, and then finally closes with the *M*. Via the progression through this full sequence, the *aum* literally embraces the whole frequency range used in human speech.

This three syllable *aum* is associated with a wealth of metaphysical meanings. Among other associations, the three syllables are associated with the Hindu trinity of Brahma-Vishnu-Shiva. In this case, the *A* sound is associated with Brahma (the creative principle), the *U* with Vishnu (the preserving principle), and *M* with Shiva (the transcendental "death" principle of transformation). Thus, the literal pronunciation of the mantra symbolizes the entire cycle of creation and manifestation. *Aum* can also be interpreted as embodying the three different planes of consciousness in which *A* is waking consciousness, *U* is dream consciousness, and *M* is the consciousness of deep sleep. In Tibetan Buddhism, *aum* represents the triad of body, mind, and voice.

Body represents all that is physical. Mind represents all that is subtle. Voice represents the coordination of the two.

And on that note, we'll leave it at that for *aum*! For one could indeed write an entire voluminous book on the meanings of this one single-syllable mantra. *Aum* presents perhaps the ultimate example of how vast amounts of information and consciousness can be encoded on one simple sound. The chanting of this seemingly simple sound may be one of the most profound practices for energetic balancing in order to establish contact with one's own creative source and higher self.

Om Gum Ganapatayei Namaha

Pronunciation: OM GUM GUH-NUH-TUH-YEI NAHM-AH-HA

This mantra serves as an honoring invocation of Ganesha, who is one of the most popular and beloved deities in the Hindi pantheon. Devotion to Ganesha is widespread throughout India and beyond, and he is worshipped by many sects in spite of other differences in their basic beliefs and affiliations. The energy form of Ganesha has universal appeal, and his primary mantra is well suited for practitioners from many backgrounds.

Ganesha is easily recognized by his large elephant head and rounded pot-bellied figure. He is often pictured in either a seated form or as a nimbly dancing figure. The free-flowing, graceful energy of this seemingly incongruous latter image hints at the main association for this deity. Ganesha is primarily revered as the remover of obstacles, the lord of good fortune, and the lord of beginnings. His mantra is often recited at the start of various ceremonies and as a blessing for any new venture of undertaking. Ganesha is also hailed as the patron of arts and sciences, the lord of letters and learning, and an archetype to assist all manifestations of creativity, intellect, and wisdom.

The energy of the Ganesha mantra is a perfect invocation to perform with the intention of removing any obstacles that may stand in the way of your goals or projects, whether they may be internal or external, psychological or physical. Along with the removal of obstacles, this mantra also invokes the blessing of good fortune, infusing your work with graceful power and powerful grace.

Om Mani Padme Hum

Pronunciation: OM MAH-NEE PAHD-MEY HOOM (Sanskrit version) or OM MAH-NEE PEY-MEY HUNG (Tibetan version)

Another one of the most well-known mantras is the *Om Mani Padme Hum* chant. This phrase can be translated as "hail the jewel in the center of the lotus." However, not unlike *om*, this mantra has a vast array of possible meanings and nuances. The chant is associated with the deity known as the Avalokitesvara, or the Buddha of Infinite Compassion, who is also known as Chenresig in the Tibetan tradition. This Buddha is visualized in the heart center as a beautiful being who holds in his hands the indestructible jewel, the lotus, and prayer beads. The Dalai Lama is said to be an incarnation of Chenresig.

The *Om Mani Padme Hum* chant unites the great mysteries of Tibetan Buddhism relating to body, speech, and mind. In essence, the heart, the throat, and the third eye/

crown are all activated with this chant. In one possible analysis of the syllables, the *om* invokes the experience of the mystery of the universal body. The *mani*, which translates as the "jewel," awakens psychic consciousness of inner vision and inspiration. *Mani* is the symbol of the highest value within our mind. In the *Padme*, which means "lotus," is experienced the mystery of the all-transforming mind. It is the symbol of spiritual unfoldment where the *mani* is finally reached. In the *hum* is experienced the synthesis of all three mysteries. Like *om*, this final syllable is untranslatable, but may be perceived as standing for the infinite within the finite.

The major significance of the *Om Mani Padme Hum* chant is its particularly powerful effectiveness in eliciting states of compassion and understanding for others. It is not typically conceived of as a mantra to resonate specific energy centers, but rather to invoke the essence of the Buddha of Infinite Compassion within one's own being. Nonetheless, there does often seem to be the activation of the heart, throat, and crown resulting from this chant. While the Tibetan Buddhists traditionally do an incredible amount of visualization while reciting this chant, the pure chanting of the mantra alone seems to be very effective in creating a field of energy that is filled with love, compassion, and understanding. This generation of heart-centered energy may be one of the most powerful benefits of any mantra, both when projected toward others and, perhaps more importantly, when accepted back in the form of self-appreciation and forgiveness toward oneself.

Exercise: Mantra Practice

As with other sound practices discussed in this book, the real understanding of mantra does not come from studying the meaning of the phrases but by immersing yourself in the pure energy of the aspects of the sound current they embody. In surrendering to the repetition of mantras with pure focus on the sounds, the mind is entrained into a deep state of meditation, free from the scattered winds of thought that can be generated by daily distractions. The mind becomes calmer, quieter, and more focused on present moment awareness. This stillness opens the gateway to receive the full current of energy invoked by the mantra.

In order to practice these mantras, first find a space where you will not be disturbed. In traditional Vedic practice, mantras are typically chanted in cycles of 108 repetitions. If you wish, a mala bead necklace can be a simple tool to assist with mantra counting. Malas are basically Tibetan prayer beads. Properly constructed malas consist of 108 beads and are available in many spiritual gift shops. However, you do not necessarily need to be concerned with this formality. In lieu of a mala, one could simply set a timer. To perform 108 repetitions of a moderate length mantra typically takes roughly five minutes. So you may simply wish to set the timer in five-minute increments depending on how long you wish to practice.

To begin, perform the type of rhythmic breathing we have used to set up previous toning sessions. But in this case, pay particular attention to establishing a feel for a particular rhythm that you will maintain throughout the practice session. A moderate rhythm in alignment with your heartbeat is often a good choice. The even pacing of the syllables of the mantras will be of value in the practice.

When you are ready, simply begin to chant your chosen mantra. You will use your normal speaking voice, but as you proceed you will quickly get a feel for a type of speak-sing approach that will serve to give the mantra more of an intonation-type quality. The exact approach will vary depending on the cadence of the mantra with which you are working.

Chant your mantra for the length of time you have predetermined. At the end of your session, allow time to sit in silence and continue to feel the vibrations of the mantra resonating both in the energy field of your being and your surrounding space. When you feel complete, stand up and perform grounding techniques as you have performed in previous sessions.

You may repeat this approach using a different mantra at another time. But we would recommend allowing a generous amount of time between mantra sessions. Ideally wait until a new day in order to allow time for the energetics of the mantra to continue to resonate. Take notice of how your experience of daily life and activities may shift and change after invoking the energy of a mantra. After engaging in another, take note of how the resonant aftereffects of different mantras create varying shifts in your experience.

Sonic Sigils

There is great value in practicing traditional mantras. It's a vast field of study that can yield rich rewards. But we would now like to introduce a technique that will allow you to create your own personal "words of power." The method borrows from the magickal practice of sigil creation. As we have noted previously, the main powers of manifestation seem to lie in the unconscious mind. The trick is to get the conscious mind, with all of its doubts and fears, out of the way so that the subconscious can fully activate.

Everyone has experienced a simple example of this process. Think of a time when you could not remember something, perhaps a name. In that sort of case, you may struggle consciously to recall whatever was forgotten. The conscious effort often results in failure to recall. But then, perhaps hours later, after you had given up consciously trying, the forgotten name spontaneously pops back into your mind. This phenomenon represents an everyday example of the unconscious mind delivering a result after it had been consciously forgotten.

On a related note, one difficulty with the practice of affirmations seems to be that they trigger resistance from the conscious mind. The technique of sigil creation is a method of representing one's affirmation in a symbolic form. The goal is then to consciously forget about it and let the unconscious work independently to accomplish your intention.

The usage of various symbols, seals, and glyphs features prominently throughout the history of magick. Indeed, there are many sizeable texts that expound on a vast array of complex iconologies from different schools in the Western esoteric tradition ranging from medieval grimoires to more modern compilations. While these images may well still have potency in an analogous fashion to how mantras may tap into the resonant waveform embodied by the chants, the modern practice of sigils takes a different approach.

Sigil magick was pioneered by the English artist and esoteric practitioner Austin Osman Spare. Spare's system involved techniques that did not rely on the study of old, traditional symbols, but rather the creation of purely individualistic images that are imbued with direct personal significance and relevance. Spare's innovations provided crucial inspiration for the modern schools of magick that advocate more personalized psychological approaches free from older superstitions and dogma. In this method of working, there is not concern over whether or not one's sigil is "correct." The primary goal is to create for yourself an image that is charged with meaning for you and you alone.

Sigil Creation

The first step in creating a sigil is to form a statement of one's desire or intent. The phrase should begin with an affirmative declaration such as "It is my desire to …" or "It is my will to …." Pick an opening declaration that feels good to you. "It is my will" seems more commanding and emphatic, but "It is my desire" could be appropriate in certain circumstances. But above all, the statement should always be phrased as a positive intention, not as a negative statement such as "It is my wish to *not experience* X" or "It is my will to *avoid* X." It has been said that the unconscious mind does not understand negative statements, therefore an affirmation phrased with a "not" statement will actually end up affirming and energizing a resonance of attraction for what you are trying to avoid!

For our example we will use the simple statement "It is my will to be healthy and happy." The overall process of creating a sigil basically involves transforming the statement of intention into a purely symbolic representation and forgetting its literal meaning. The first step is to write your sentence out in all capital letters:

IT IS MY WILL TO BE HEALTHY AND HAPPY

Next, go through the sentence and cross out any duplicate letters. (Note: Some sources for sigil instruction also advise removing the vowels. We like to keep the vowels due to the powerful energetic elements contained in these sounds.)

I T I̶ S M Y W I̶ L̶ L̶ T̶ O B E H E̶ A̶ L̶ T̶ H̶ Y̶ A̶ N D H̶ A̶ P P̶ Y̶

In this case, you will be left with the letters

I T S M Y W L O B E H A N D P

The primary traditional sigil method would be to take these letters and form them into a symbolic glyph. Note that this is a purely creative process and there is no right or wrong way. The best approach is to relax and go into a light meditative state and simply look at the shapes of the letters. Then assemble them into an abstract design such as this:

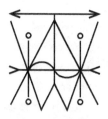

Sample Sigil

To create such a symbol, first try to incorporate all the letters in your image, and then feel free to shift them around, write them backward or upside down, and keep an eye out for places where already existing lines and angles may imply other letters. Then clean it up a little and add little stylistic garnishes until you end up with a design that feels impactful to you. In doing so, know that the essence of your original statement is now symbolically represented in a more highly condensed, encoded fashion.

After you are happy with your creation, the next task is to activate and charge the sigil in such a way that the image, along with its meaning, is implanted in the unconscious. The traditional process involves ritualistically internalizing the sigil while in an energized or altered state. After that step, you are to banish the sigil from your conscious mind and forget it so that the unconscious can obey the encoded instructions without being hindered by afterthoughts. For full details about visual sigil creation, please see the book by Frater U. D. in the recommended resources section. We will focus here on how to accomplish this result with sound.

Creating Sonic Sigils

Instead of the ritually charged visual sigils described above, we are instead going to use a comparable method in order to create personal words of power or mantras. This method is purely creative, and once again, there is no right or wrong. The key is to relax, have fun with the process, and tap into your intuitive, creative guidance.

The first steps in this method are the same as with the visual sigil method above. First formulate a statement of intention. To begin, we will use the same sentence "It is my will to be healthy and happy." Then, as before, remove all duplicate letters. Which yielded

ITSMYWLOBEHANDP

Now the fun part begins. To create a sonic sigil simply take the remaining letters and use them to create a new word or phrase. You could use the letters in the existing order, but it may be more effective to scramble them up into a new, even more unrecognizable sequence. From what we have to work with above, one possibility could be

DHANTWILSBEPOMY

From there, simply play with different articulations of the new phrase, pronouncing it phonetically with accents in various places until you settle on a chant with a good satisfying rhythm. One possible pronunciation of the letters above could be *DAAHN-TWILLS-BEPO-MEYE*. Once again, there is no right or wrong way. It's your own unique creation!

Exercise: Sonic Sigil Practice

Once you have settled on your new phrase, you may use it in the same fashion as traditional mantras. The first time you practice with your sonic sigil, find yourself a quiet place where you will not be disturbed. Settle into a comfortable, upright posture and begin to do some energized, rhythmic breathing as we have done in previous exercises. After a few moments, begin to chant your phrase. Repeat it over and over until you begin to forget what the original sentence was that you used to construct it. Perhaps you can recall the childhood game where you repeated a word over and over until it began to sound like nonsense? That's the goal here as well.

Repeat your sonic sigil until it sounds like meaningless babble, and know that the more you forget its literal meaning, the more your chosen statement of intention will be seeded into the unconscious mind. Continue chanting for as long as it feels appropriate. When you are done, sit in a state of silent meditation for several moments. After that, stand up, ground yourself, and reset your energy field with a burst of laughter and body movement. Then go do something fun and distracting that will allow you to forget all about your sigil practice. On follow-up workings after the sigil has been charged by this initial session, feel free to repeat your phrase anytime, anywhere, for as long as you desire in order to revive and recirculate the energy of your intention.

Alternate Sonic Sigil Method

Before we move on from this topic, we would like to offer an additional simplified method for sonic sigil creation. This method can be done spontaneously in any setting. Rather than creating a full sentence statement and analytically crossing out the letters, simply form a list of qualities or conditions you would like to experience or attract. One possible application could perhaps be to transmute a certain emotion that is causing you difficulty.

For example, imagine that you have to do a public presentation or performance that you are feeling nervous or fearful about. That emotion of fear can cast an aura of unpleasantness about the upcoming task. In order to transmute what you are feeling, first think of a list of qualities that embody the opposite of the emotion you would like to transmute. To accomplish this process, it's useful to first tap into the states you would like to experience as simple sensations of feeling or energy flow in the body. In the case of fear, it's interesting to note that the body sensation of fear, especially as triggered by ruminations about an upcoming unfamiliar experience, is basically the same as the feeling of anticipation or excitement. It's only the attachment of the defining emotional label of *fear* to the sensation that causes it to become unpleasant.

The first step in the transmutation process is to create a list of the qualities that embody what you would like to feel in the upcoming situation. For the purpose of our example, the list could perhaps be "adventure, excitement, fun, and anticipation."

Once you have the list, simply take one of the prominent syllables or prominent groups of letters from each word. One possible result from our sample list could be "AD EX FU ANT." Pronounce the syllables as a new word—*Adexfuant*. Perform the initial charging of your sonic sigil as per the method described above. But in future usage, imagine yourself mentally rehearsing or stepping into the situation that you used to feel fearful about. Chant your sonic sigil of transmutation while evoking all of the positive feeling embodied by your list of words. As you do so, feel that former feeling of fear being transmuted into its opposite.

Step Into a World of Magick

We hope you have enjoyed these brief tastes of the worlds of magick and mantra. As we have noted, the art and science of these disciplines comprise vast fields of study. But some of the works in the recommended resources section will set your feet on a good path. And note that certain topics discussed in the more esoteric dimensions of these fields may seem highly unusual at first. But if you keep a balanced approach tempered with healthy skepticism, many adventures could await you in these powerful arenas. Furthermore, the additional awareness of sound and vibration we are trying to encourage may well yield insights that are only hinted at in the various texts. After all, the word *occult* simply means "hidden." Take one step at a time, and know that ultimately all of the topics and phenomena discussed in magick are merely aspects and extensions of your own vast consciousness!

Recommended Reading

Healing Mantras: Using Sound Affirmations for Personal Power, Creativity, and Healing by Thomas Ashley-Farrand

Mantra Yoga and Primal Sound: Secrets of Seed (Bija) Mantras by David Frawley

Words of Power: Sacred Sounds of East & West by Brian Crowley and Esther Crowley

The Yoga of Sound: Tapping the Hidden Power of Music and Chant by Russill Paul

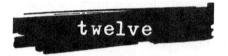

twelve

The World Symphony:
Group Toning and Global Healing

The true sound of healing is love.

—SARAH "SARUAH" BENSON

Throughout this book we have explored various approaches for working with sound on an individual level to gain an understanding of the basic power of vibration to create energetic shift and change in the laboratory of your own experience. But to take it all to the next level, we would like to encourage and inspire you to explore the power of sound within the larger frame of group work.

When we make sound with others, the processes of entrainment and resonance become quickly evident. As a group tones, people enter into a state of enhanced coherence. This coherent resonance begins to happen almost immediately, but it increases the longer the group tones together. The effect is also amplified by intentionality. When the group is toning with a shared intention, there is a powerful feeling of unity. Group toning offers unique insights about the nature of co-created reality while also being a great deal of fun.

This type of working may be one of the most powerful callings in these times. No one would deny that there are many problematic issues and conditions that need to be addressed in our modern world. Indeed, the continued survival of our current civilization may depend on the urgent actions of the next generation or two. As much as we are great believers in all of the esoteric aspects and applications of sound work, a crucial measuring stick of any energy healing modality is "how does it help to improve daily life on a practical level?" and by extension "how does it benefit the well-being of all the inhabitants of the planet?"

As we have discussed in various ways throughout this book, the energy of sound forms a unified field between the subtle energy realm and the physical plane. Applications of sound work can be found in many seemingly separate modalities, and the awareness of the basic principles of sound can yield insights that will enhance understanding and effectiveness in all of these realms of practice. Similarly, sound can also form powerful bonds and bridges between people, serving to enhance a greater unity of consciousness and collective intelligence.

Mystics and spiritual teachers throughout the ages have been pointing the way toward greater unity of humankind. But one of the more powerful modern encapsulations of this outlook was put forth in the mid-twentieth century by the French Jesuit priest Pierre Teilhard de Chardin, who once proposed that "we are ... moving forward toward some new critical point that lies ahead, a harmonized collectivity of consciousness equivalent to a sort of super-consciousness."[30]

Teilhard de Chardin was one of the main proponents of the concept of the noosphere. This term derives from the Greek words *nous*, which means "mind" and *sphaira*, meaning "sphere." The noosphere could be thought of as a type of mental (or mind) sheath that encompasses the planet and all of its biological and environmental systems. The philosophy of the noosphere proposes the evolution of a coherent field of consciousness and collective intelligence, which, among other things, will eventually attain the power to influence and reshape the biosphere of the basic physical conditions on Earth. Various other thinkers have also contributed to the development of this philosophy and the ideas have informed the popular beliefs that have emerged in the mind/body/spirit communities regarding the global brain and Gaia consciousness.

While these thoughts may merely seem like lofty, impractical mysticism at first, there has been a growing amount of evidence in the past couple decades to support the validity of the power of collective intelligence, as well as various organizations supporting the development of a collective wisdom movement. Notable contributors to this field include the Global Consciousness Project, the Institute of Noetic Sciences, the Collective Wisdom Initiative, and the Global Leadership Initiative, whose mission statement is nothing less than to

---

30. Robert Kenny, "The Science of Collective Consciousness," in *What Is Enlightenment: Redefining Spirituality for an Evolving World* (May 1, 2004): 78.

generate a tipping point in humanity's ability to address its most critical global challenges.

This concept of collective intelligence also has its roots in the work of the visionary scientist Rupert Sheldrake, who first proposed the concept of morphogenetic fields. The theory of morphogenetic fields is an intricate and nuanced concept, but in the simplest nutshell they are basically fields of thought and structures of consciousness that permeate and influence all existence. These fields are subtle patterns of energy on higher levels of organization and creation that may ultimately be responsible for the multitude of manifestations on the physical plane. We have already explored the power of sound to create and shape form and energetic fields. Now the task is to apply it all on a more expansive, practical level.

Group Coherence Research

While the dreams of a great collective intelligence are all inspiring to contemplate, one can't help but raise the obvious question "Is it all real?" It appears that many people are fascinated by this question, for there has been a surge of interest in recent decades toward determining and measuring the effects of group coherence. This multidisciplinary work seems to indicate that the answer is "Yes!" Some of the original and most influential of these studies were conducted by practitioners of Transcendental Meditation (TM). Via a series of social experiments that began in the 1970s, the TM organization, and its offshoot TM-Siddhi Program, set out to prove that groups of meditators could create a coherent field of consciousness that has beneficial effects on surrounding communities. The experiments were initially conducted in eleven cities in the United States with many positive results, such as reduced crime rate, decreased suicide rate, and even a reduction in the number of automobile accidents![31]

This phenomenon became known as the Maharishi Effect, named after TM founder Maharishi Mahesh Yogi. One of the thought-provoking conclusions was that the beneficial results could be achieved when only 1 percent of a given community engaged in the meditation practices. This is an extraordinary claim, for it was further predicted that a group with size equal to the square root of 1 percent of a population would have a measurable influence on the quality of life. For example, a group of 200 practicing focused meditation together in a city of four million (100 x 200 x 200) would be sufficient to influence the whole city. Furthermore, based on the population estimates at the time of the first studies, it was speculated that a group of 1,600 would be capable of affecting the whole United States, and a mere 7,000 worldwide would be able to influence the entire global population!

Here we have a very inspiring thought form, especially considering that many of the messages we receive via various media channels seem to be intended to keep us all in a fear-based state of helplessness. What if it were true that such a relatively small group could indeed shift the frequencies of the entire planet? Then the actions and vibrations of each individual take on new significance. For no matter where

---

31. Maharishi Programmes, "Maharishi Effect Research," accessed February 14, 2015. http://maharishi-programmes .globalgoodnews.com/maharishi-effect/research.html.

we are, we can all contribute toward the tipping point of the global field.

As intriguing as their work is, the TM groups are not the only contributors to the field of group coherence. Noteworthy research is also being conducted by such groups as the Global Consciousness Project (GCP) out of the University of Princeton. Rather than examining sociological data, the GCP uses random number generators to measure fluctuations in group consciousness. These number generators produce random output of ones and zeros, so their activity could basically be thought of as an elaborate series of coin tosses. In standard operation, the results are more or less fifty-fifty. However, the essence of the GCP research indicates that during periods of increased collective attention or emotion the number generators produce results that are significantly less random and begin to follow more orderly patterns. These deviations from pure chance are noted worldwide through a global network of physical random number generators, thus demonstrating a nonlocal effect. It is also interesting to note that results are enhanced depending on the type of event being measured. For example, events such as large-scale sports games, even though they may be charged with high degrees of public attention and emotion, do not produce as orderly a pattern as smaller groups of people performing activities with more direct conscious focus. So it seems that the quality of consciousness involved is a greater factor than the sheer energy generated by an event. Activities involving more active intention produce greater coherence in the collective field than passive entertainment spectacles.

In spite of encouraging initial results, this work is still in its infancy. It will be exciting to see how it all continues to develop, for this contemplation of the power of collective consciousness seems like a logical extension of the evolution of human thought. Conventional science began with the contemplation of the physical world and material processes. It then evolved to embrace the existence of finer gravitational, electric, and magnetic fields. The current emergence of interest in and study of subtle energy represents the next evolution to finer bandwidths of energetic manifestation. It's likely that future generations will regard the existence of subtle energy as being as self-evident as our current regard of gravity. But the concept of collective consciousness may be the ultimate plateau of consideration, for as we have noted in various ways in previous chapters, the creative field of consciousness may be the ultimate driving force that fuels all creation and manifestation.

There is a wealth of rapidly growing documentation of the validity of the effects of collective intelligence. But if these concepts sound far-fetched to anyone, note that as recently in the evolution of human understanding as the 1700s the concept of meteorites was denounced as vehemently as the UFO phenomenon is scorned in certain mainstream scientific circles today. The existence of meteorites is now accepted as a grade school scientific fact. Every generation that has believed itself to have the final word in scientific understanding has proven to be wrong. Our current generation will be no exception!

Rather than continue to contemplate the phenomenon of group intelligence philosophically, we would like to simply offer some ways in which you may begin to experience it yourself. Once again, sound and vocal toning can be the forces that will open the gateway, for the first initiation can come via simply assembling a group of people to make sound. As we first tune our own instruments with personal sound work and then bring people together into harmonious groups, the more we will be able to contribute melodies to a greater global symphony of consciousness.

How to Start a Toning Group

In all likelihood there may not be an active sound work or toning group in your area. How can you start up a toning group? The basic first task is to do whatever it takes to bring people together! You do not have to have mastered all of the topics we've discussed in this book to get started. As you will quickly discover as you proceed, the process of sounding quickly evokes a sense of higher group intelligence that will help guide your proceedings. Simply gathering people to make sound together is enough.

Also note that you don't necessarily need many people. Group toning works with any number of people from two up. More is not necessarily better, but a group of twenty has very different energy than a group of five. Regardless of numbers, the sonic alchemy of a toning group is different every time. Any changes to the multiple variables associated with the group will have notable effects. Such changes could be the addition of new personalities or a change in the group intentionality. The group sound will be also be affected by the members' expectations and emotions, which, interestingly enough, could in turn shift during the course of the toning.

Before we offer our model, note that a toning group could be a very simple affair. Our typical toning group meeting usually lasts roughly an hour and a half. Before taking on that commitment, you could perhaps introduce the practice as part of a social gathering of like-minded people. All you have to do is describe the concept of what you would like to do, and then simply begin making sound together! Any of the exercises listed throughout this book could provide a starting point, and a session of ten to fifteen minutes could be enough to trigger new interest in the activity. If you would like to proceed further, below is an outline of approaches that have worked well for us, but know that they could well be subject to change depending on the actual dynamics of your group. Take the elements that are helpful for you, but be like the sound current itself, flexible and adaptive.

Open with Sound

First of all, be patient with yourself and others; making sound in public requires some bravery. Although we have noted that toning is different in style and purpose from performance singing, it can initially bring up the same anxieties in many people, particularly in a group setting. You can help alleviate these anxieties by creating a comfortable space and encouraging playfulness. Let the group know they can experiment with sound without judgments. Making tones together is not about performing, but rather about expressing energy in a collective form with others. Once we can let go of the limitations of trying to sound "good," we'll all be astounded by the sort of tones that come through us within a group setting.

When we begin a session, even before basic introductions, we like to make an immediate sound together for a few minutes. The only instruction you should offer at this point is that the sound should be allowed to roll in a freeform fashion, which is to say that each person should tone in his or her own comfortable breath cycle. This style will permit everyone's individual tones to overlap and interweave, not merely end up as a group unison tone where everyone starts and stops together. This primary tone starts to form the group coherent field and begins the process of group mind entrainment. This first tone should be something simple and universal, such as an *ah* sound or an *om*.

The *ah* sound is useful because it lacks any connection to any specific spiritual tradition. Any sounds that you choose to use will depend on the open-mindedness of your own group. However, we believe that all sounds regardless of tradition can be utilized, and most people will be comfortable, as long the sounds are presented in a respectful, non-dogmatic fashion. That is, we acknowledge and honor the sacred nature of any given sound without requiring others to do the same. In general, one of the great strengths of sound work is that it is not tied to any singular tradition, yet can be engaged in from within the framework of any tradition. Of course, there are certain soundings and mantras associated with particular traditions, but the general use of sound work belongs to everyone, and thus can be claimed to belong solely to no one.

Group Introductions

After the initial sound, you can introduce yourself and talk a little about the purpose of the group. For us, a primary purpose of group toning is simply to spread the experience of sound. We always like to remind ourselves to keep talking to a minimum, though. It is important to communicate directions and information, but we like to spend as much time as possible in the state of actual toning. From our experience, our purpose is usually best met by allowing the experiential nature of sound work to take the participants on their own unique journeys of discovery with minimal preconditioning of expectations. Simply providing people with the space to explore the power of sound in a group will impart many of the greatest teachings of sound without words.

Next we like to go around the group and have each participant state their name and a simple intention they would like to focus on for themselves during the toning group. This procedure serves to let each individual be heard and recognized while simultaneously beginning to cord them further into the co-created group energy. For the sake of simplicity, it is useful to go first as a demonstration for the group and to set the complexity of intentionality. We suggest keeping the intention to a single word such as *patience* or *acceptance*, or perhaps a simple phrase such as "going with the flow" or "inner peace." These basic intentions are useful not only because they keep the exercise moving along quickly, but also because simplicity and clarity are helpful for maintaining focus on the intention.

First Toning Session: Personal Intentions

At this point before beginning the first group tone, we like to inform the group that we will be in state of silence for a few minutes after each tone ends. We highlight quickly that that state of silence is important for allowing the shifts from the tone to settle and take effect. Then we proceed to leading the group in the first free-form toning session. Remind people to tone in the same sort of rolling fashion as we did with the introductory sound. For this first session, we like to focus on the personal level, inviting each participant to focus on the intention they expressed earlier.

The free-form toning usually lasts between ten and twenty minutes. If the tone is much longer or shorter, it is our advice to allow it to be. The tones often seem to have a mind of their own. We like to ring a pair of Tibetan bells to indicate the beginning and end of the sounding. This is not necessary, but it is helpful to add a small level of ceremony for participants to frame the sound experience.

We often begin the session in near silence, simply making breath sounds on the exhale, and then we slowly build into a hum. From the hum we expand into open voice tones, which could be various vowel sounds, wordless syllables, overtones, and whatever tones we feel energized to create. The Immersion into Sound exercise described in chapter 6 can also serve as a good model for how to guide participants from silence into sound.

Interlude: Group Exercises

After the first free-form toning session, we like to pause for reflection and invite participants to share any thoughts or comments. Then we usually like to present a structured teaching session or activity. We may sometimes teach and lead a group chant of a specific mantra during this time. Both of these change-ups offer a nice contrast from the spontaneous, improvisational nature of free-form tonings.

Once again, any of the exercises presented throughout this book could be applied or adapted to a group experience, for as you continue to practice them yourself, insights will inevitably come regarding how they may be shared with others. This interlude activity often takes another fifteen or twenty minutes, depending on the complexity of the chosen sound exercise. But note that this phase is optional. If you wish, you may choose to skip the division into two sessions and remain in pure tone for your entire gathering without breaking for other activities or discussion until the end.

In any case, after this halfway point it's advisable to take a quick stretch and movement break.

Second Toning Session: Planetary Intentions

After the break, we then begin a second rolling free-form toning session. This time we expand the focus from the personal level to the planetary level. We always find the changes that naturally occur for this secondary free-form toning session interesting. You too may find that this second toning session often sounds more harmonious and seems more unified in nature. Is this because the intention changed focus from personal to planetary? Or is it a natural function of having spent more time in sound together and therefore coming into a greater state of resonance? We believe it to be a little bit of both. In any case, as before, we ring the Tibetan bells and begin to tone.

This second toning session typically lasts another fifteen to twenty minutes. And afterward, as before, we take a period of silence followed by some time for reflection. We ask for any questions or comments about the toning experience. This is also a good chance to remind the group of the next meeting time or promote any future gatherings before you end the session. And finally, to wrap it all up, we always like to end with a final grounding group tone, which we like to refer to as "the *om* to go home."

Toning Group Overview

And there we have it! A basic model for a possible approach to conducting a toning group. What has happened here? We'd like to offer a quick overview analysis in light of various concepts we've presented throughout this book. We've talked about how you can self-entrain. You can change your heart rhythms, brain waves, and frequency patterns with self-created sound. What happens when we work with sound in groups is that the members entrain with one another. The entrainment happens on biological and emotional levels. Most importantly, it can happen on the level of intentionality. When we entrain our intentions together, their potency greatly rises. Imagine small currents in the ocean joining to create massive waves.

Group entrainment begins automatically when we make sound together. In fact, it would be quite difficult not to entrain with others when toning in a group. You would have to actively try not to entrain, and even then you would be entraining in your intentionality of not entraining. Conformity in nonconformity, as it were. Regardless, we generally are trying to actively entrain together when group toning. The good news is that this benefit does not require conscious effort, for group coherence starts on its own. The better news is that not only is the process naturally spontaneous whenever a group makes sound together, it can also be aided via the synergy of conscious intent.

We recommended earlier that when working with a group it is helpful to make a sound together right off the bat. This initial sound both literally and figuratively sets the tone for the group. We then recommended having everyone in the group state their name and a personal intention. The name is important because it is a personalized mantra. Our names are words of power that we use every day casually, but they are tremendously important. Remember the old folk tales in which knowing the true name of a magical creature could give you power over it? Our names are powerful. They are the sounds by which we introduce ourselves to the world.

The act of each person putting forth a personal intention may initially seem counterproductive to producing a coherent unified field. But in fact the inclusion of differing personalized intents can be extremely useful in creating the group coherence. There are a few reasons for this. First off, allowing everyone to add his or her personal intention invests the individual participant's energy into the group connection. Additionally, the individualized intentions have a way of spreading throughout the group via energetic resonance. That is to say that just because someone's intention is individual doesn't mean it won't become a group intention. The individual intentions do merge into larger unified group intentions, and it's interesting that many times the intentions of the various individuals often run along the same theme.

From there, the actual tonings take on a life of their own, which sprouts from the collective dynamic of any given group. The volume of the group sound may rise and fall, and the dynamics may shift and change as certain voices may rise to prominence and then fade to the background. Spontaneous melodies may emerge, and periods of beautiful harmonization may arise contrasting with phases of dissonance. In this sense, the toning group can be a mirror for life itself. But, through the power of sound, the end result is always a return to harmonious unity. We have never had a toning session that has ended on a sour note.

Future Possibilities for Group Sound Work

Can group sound work apply to situations outside of a toning group? Long story short, just as many small streams can make a great river and a powerful wave is created by individual droplets of water, we feel that the potential exists in any situation when large numbers of people are gathered together. In fact, a group energy field is already created whenever crowds come together.

For example, imagine you're at a concert standing right in front of the stage surrounded by a large audience. You don't personally know anyone around you, but you feel connected to them nonetheless. The music you're all listening to creates a shared sense of emotion. Now most all of us can relate to this sort of experience, but what if this sense of connection was coupled with a shared purpose? A purpose shared not just by those listening to the music, but also by those creating the music. This action blurs the line between performer and listener, making the listeners active participants in manifesting a shared collective vision.

In recent years, there has been an explosion in the popularity of various types of music festivals ranging from affairs with multiple live bands to assorted electronic dance music acts. We can't help but wonder if this phenomenon is a reflection of a collective desire for unification via music and sound in and of itself. These festivals offer great potential for the unification of sound and conscious intent that could be directed toward positive global change. Even though the main motive of attendees at these events is simply to have a fun, joyous experience, that alone is a strong starting platform of collective intent. In fact, it is perhaps ideal, for projecting intentionality on sound is most powerful when it comes from a place of happiness and bliss.

Even if the end goal of using sound to affect positive change on a large level is a serious intent, the ways and means of getting to the goal should not be taken as a solemn duty. Even the Bible says "Make a joyful noise unto the Lord." Remember laughter is perhaps one of the most powerful forms of toning, available naturally and spontaneously to us all. Sacred and solemn are not synonymous!

That being said, a medium ground must be found if the events are to move beyond mere amusement platforms. Shared enthusiasm and positivity alone are not enough if the end goal is to be more than just entertainment. For example, a few years ago Joshua attended an MC Yogi concert to see and experience what was being done in the field of positive, conscious music. MC Yogi offered songs that combined positive hip-hop lyrics, Sanskrit mantras, and electronic dance beats. The crowd was enthusiastic and engaged during the songs and would often sing along with the chants. The presence of amplified heart energy was filling the theater. However, at one point in between songs, MC Yogi attempted to engage the audience in a more interactive exercise. But the buzz in the theater was for the most part too loud; people chatted with their neighbors and sipped their drinks.

The performer attempted to gather the crowd's focus with the words "class is in session." But it was to little avail. Some people engaged in what MC Yogi was trying to initiate, but for the most part members of the crowd were chatting amongst themselves waiting for the next song to start. This is not to say that those people who just wanted to enjoy themselves were incorrect in their actions. They were doing exactly what they were used to, which was being part of a passive audience waiting to be entertained. There is nothing wrong with this! But if we wish to use the power of sound to influence change on the large group level, we must move past the audience and entertainer paradigm.

Music festivals and large concert events have tremendous potential to utilize the combined powers of group energy dynamics and internationalized sound to create great positive change in the world. The performers onstage will do what they can do to guide and initiate the proceedings, but each member of the crowd must also accept and honor their own role as a vital part of an energetic orchestra of consciousness. The featured performer can serve a vital role as conductor of the group energy, but the true power emanates from the keynotes of personal vibration offered by each unique individual. This great power and responsibility could be extended to our role as citizens of Earth, which is the greatest concert hall of all! Here we are not only all members of the audience, but we also all have awesome potential to be composer, conductor, and performer all in one.

Coda

We thank you for joining us in the journey through the world of sound. We're covered a lot of ground. We appreciate the time and attention you have shared with us. Over the course of this book we have explored crucial building block fundamentals of toning and sound work, and we have also looked at more targeted sound exercises relating to energy work. We have used sound to tone the elemental energy centers related to the five elements: earth, water, fire, air, and ether. We have resonated the energy centers with vowel tonings and elemental bija mantras.

We have also spontaneously generated our own tones for the five elements based on intuitive associations. We even discovered the powerful energetics of natural, spontaneous body sounds and offered some thoughts on how sound can be used as a tool for personal manifestation. It is our deepest intent that through these exercises and interactions with sound you have gained insights into the more subtle modalities of vibration that go beyond what mere words can express.

We've touched on a wide array of different disciplines, but, as we've often noted, have only revealed the tip of the iceberg of all of them. Yet we hope that we have demonstrated that the energy of sound forms a connective thread between all of them. *Nada brahma!*

If we have offered any new insights or inspired you to adopt any new practices or pursue any new fields of study, then we will have fulfilled our purpose. But above all, we encourage you to continue exploring the experiential sound work exercises we have presented! Make them your own and create your own variations. As we have often stressed, direct experience with the vibrant, living sound current will always be your most powerful teacher.

Above all, always keep in mind that the highest purpose of all these studies and practices is to assist in the evolution of consciousness and intelligence on the planet. And, in doing so, we will hopefully improve the ways in which we all treat one another. As you proceed on these paths, also recall that the highest power is always achieved via the heart-centered waveforms of love and service. For just as Earth supports our lives, the vibrations we feed back to the field of the planet serve to nourish our shared energy field. Therefore, the question we should always be asking ourselves on an ongoing basis is "What am I feeding the field?"

The epigraph for this chapter comes from one of the great influential teachers in the field of sound healing, and Joshua's godmother, Sarah "Saruah" Benson. This simple phrase—the true sound of healing is love—is worth deep contemplation. For indeed one of the highest goals of sound and all energy work is the enhancement of love and compassion to be used in service beyond the separate self to the benefit of all beings, for sound is a unifying modality that can also be used to join the energies of people all across the globe. We have seen this potential come to life many times in workshop settings where a group of strangers comes together at the beginning and by the end become unified into an extraordinary new family and community. All it took for these new bonds to manifest was to become immersed in the power of sound. It is easy to imagine how this attunement could expand out to a global level. The powers of sound and toning are universal energy forms that can be felt and understood regardless of creed or ethnic background.

In closing, we can't help but think of the charming old song "I'd Like to Teach the World to Sing (In Perfect Harmony)." If you pause for a moment, perhaps you can begin to hear that song in your head now. How does it make you feel? Maybe there's a smile creeping onto your face. If so, good! A childlike spirit of new possibility is the first step toward new evolution. But perhaps teaching the world to tone would be a more powerful universal goal. And thus all people from all corners of the globe could sound forth together with Intonations for In-Tune-Nations. Just imagine the possibility. Now take a deep breath and sound forth...

Recommended Reading

The Field: The Quest for the Secret Force of the Universe by Lynne McTaggart

Healing Words: The Power of Prayer and the Practice of Medicine by Larry Dossey

The Intention Experiment: Using Your Thoughts to Change Your Life and the World by Lynne McTaggart

The Isaiah Effect: Decoding the Lost Science of Prayer and Prophecy by Gregg Braden

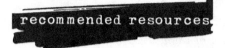

Ackerman, Diane. *A Natural History of the Senses.* New York: Random House, 1990.

Andrews, Ted. *Crystal Balls & Crystal Bowls: Tools for Ancient Scrying & Modern Seership.* St. Paul, MN: Llewellyn Publications, 1994.

———. *The Healer's Manual: A Beginner's Guide to Vibrational Therapies.* St. Paul, MN: Llewellyn Publications, 1993.

———. *Sacred Sounds: Transformation Through Music & Word.* St. Paul, MN: Llewellyn Publications, 1992.

Ashley-Farrand, Thomas. *Chakra Mantras: Liberate Your Spiritual Genius Through Chanting.* San Francisco: Red Wheel/Weiser, 2006.

———. *Healing Mantras: Using Sound Affirmations for Personal Power, Creativity, and Healing.* New York: Ballantine, 1999.

Bandler, Richard. *Richard Bandler's Guide to Trance-formation: How to Harness the Power of Hypnosis to Ignite Effortless and Lasting Change.* Deerfield Beach, FL: Health Communications, 2008.

Beaulieu, John. *Human Tuning: Sound Healing with Tuning Forks.* High Falls, NY: BioSonics Enterprises, 2010.

Berendt, Joachim-Ernst. *The Third Ear: On Listening to the World.* Shaftesbury, UK: Element, 1988.

———. *The World Is Sound: Nada Brahma: Music and the Landscape of Consciousness.* Rochester, VT: Destiny Books, 1991.

Braden, Gregg. *The Isaiah Effect: Decoding the Lost Science of Prayer and Prophecy.* New York: Harmony Books, 2000.

Brodie, Renee. *The Healing Tones of Crystal Bowls: Heal Yourself with Sound and Colour.* Vancouver: Aroma Art, 1996.

Bruyere, Rosalyn. *Wheels of Light: Charas, Auras, and the Healing Energy of the Body.* New York: Fireside, 1989.

Campbell, Don G. *The Mozart Effect: Tapping Into the Power of Music to Heal the Body, Strengthen the Mind, and Unlock the Creative Spirit.* New York: Harper, 2001.

————. *Music Physician for Times to Come: An Anthology.* Wheaton, IL: Theosophical Pub. House, 1991.

————. *The Roar of Silence: Healing Powers of Breath, Tone & Music.* Wheaton, IL: Theosophical Pub. House, 1989.

Campbell, Don G., and Alex Doman. *Healing at the Speed of Sound: How What We Hear Transforms Our Brains and Our Lives.* New York: Penguin, 2011.

Chopra, Deepak. *Quantum Healing: Exploring the Frontiers of Mind/Body Medicine.* New York: Bantam Books, 1990.

Collinge, William. *Subtle Energy: Awakening to the Unseen Forces in Our Lives.* New York: Warner Books, 1998.

Crowley, Brian, and Esther Crowley. *Words of Power: Sacred Sounds of East & West.* St. Paul, MN: Llewellyn Publications, 1991.

Cymatics. "What Is Cymatics?" Accessed March 5, 2015. www.cymatics.org.

D'Angelo, James. *The Healing Power of the Human Voice: Mantras, Chants, and Seed Sounds for Health and Harmony.* Rochester, VT: Healing Arts Press, 2005.

————. *Seed Sounds for Tuning the Chakras: Vowels, Consonants, and Syllables for Spiritual Transformation.* Rochester, VT: Destiny Books, 2012.

Dossey, Larry. *Healing Words: The Power of Prayer and the Practice of Medicine.* New York: Harper, 1997.

Frater U. D. *Practical Sigil Magic: Creating Personal Symbols for Success.* Rev. ed. Woodbury, MN: Llewellyn Publications, 2012.

Frawley, David. *Mantra Yoga and Primal Sound: Secrets of Seed (Bija) Mantras.* Twin Lakes, WI: Lotus Press, 2010.

Galgut, Peter N. *Humming Your Way to Happiness: Healing and Meditative Sounds and Overtone Singing from around the World*. New York: O Books, 2005.

Gardner, Kay. *Sounding the Inner Landscape: Music as Medicine*. Stonington, ME: Caduceus Publications, 1990.

Gardner-Gordon, Joy. *The Healing Voice: Traditional & Contemporary Toning, Chanting & Singing*. Freedom, CA: Crossing Press, 1993.

Gass, Robert, and Kathleen Brehony. *Chanting: Discovering Spirit in Sound*. New York: Broadway, 1999.

Gerber, Richard. *Vibrational Medicine: New Choices for Healing Ourselves*. Updated ed. Santa Fe, NM: Bear & Co., 1996.

Goldman, Jonathan, and Andi Goldman. *Chakra Frequencies: Tantra of Sound*. Rochester, VT: Destiny Books, 2011.

———. *The 7 Secrets of Sound Healing*. London: Hay House, 2008.

Gustafson, Eric. *The Ringing Sound: An Introduction to the Sound Current*. Austin, TX: Conscious Living Press, 2000.

Harner, Michael. "Journeywork: Shamanic Journeying Recordings." The Foundation for Shamanic Studies. www.shamanism.org/products/audio.html.

Hendricks, Gay. *Conscious Breathing: Breathwork for Health, Stress Release, and Personal Mastery*. New York: Bantam Books, 1995.

Jansen, Eva Rudy. *Singing Bowls: A Practical Handbook of Instruction and Use.* Dover, Holland: Binkey Kok Publications, 1992.

Judith, Anodea. *Wheels of Life: A User's Guide to the Chakra System.* St. Paul, MN: Llewellyn Publications, 1987.

Kenyon, Tom. *Brain States.* Lithia Springs, GA: World Tree Press, 2011.

Keyes, Laurel Elizabeth, and Don G. Campbell. *Toning: The Creative and Healing Power of the Voice.* New ed. Camarillo, CA: DeVorss, 2008.

Khan, Hazrat Inayat. *The Music of Life.* Omega Uniform ed. New Lebanon, NY: Omega Press, 1988.

———. *The Mysticism of Sound and Music.* Rev. ed. Boston: Shambhala, 1996.

Leeds, Joshua. *The Power of Sound: How to Manage Your Personal Soundscape for a Vital, Productive, and Healthy Life.* Rochester, VT: Healing Arts Press, 2001.

Levitin, Daniel J. *This Is Your Brain on Music: The Science of a Human Obsession.* New York: Dutton, 2006.

McClellan, Randall. *The Healing Forces of Music: History, Theory, and Practice.* Amity, NY: Amity House, 1988.

McTaggart, Lynne. *The Field: The Quest for the Secret Force of the Universe.* Updated ed. New York: Harper, 2008.

———. *The Intention Experiment: Using Your Thoughts to Change Your Life and the World.* New York: Free Press, 2008.

Mumford, Jonn. *A Chakra & Kundalini Workbook: Psycho-Spiritual Techniques for Health Rejuvenation, Psychic*

Powers & Spiritual Realization. 2nd rev. ed. St. Paul, MN: Llewellyn Publications, 1994.

Narby, Jeremy. *Shamans Through Time: 500 Years on the Path to Knowledge.* New York: J.P. Tarcher/Putnam, 2001.

Parker, Scott E., and Jamison A. Smith. *Musician's Acoustics.* Boulder, CO: Scott E. Parker, Jamison A. Smith, 2013.

Paul, Russill. *The Yoga of Sound: Tapping the Hidden Power of Music and Chant.* Novato, CA: New World Library, 2004.

Perret, Daniel Gilbert. *Sound Healing with the Five Elements: Sound Instruments, Sound Therapy, Sound Energy.* Dover, Holland: Binkey Kok Publications, 2005.

Rama, Swami, Rudolph Ballentine, and Alan Hymes. *Science of Breath: A Practical Guide.* Honesdale, PA: Himalayan Institute Press, 1979.

Rosen, Richard. *The Yoga of Breath: A Step-by-Step Guide to Pranayama.* Boston: Shambhala, 2002.

Sacks, Oliver. *Musicophilia: Tales of Music and the Brain.* Rev. ed. New York: Random House, 2008.

Sigil Daily. "Creation & Activation." Accessed March 5, 2015. http://sigildaily.com/activating-rituals/.

Three Initiates. *The Kybalion: A Study of the Hermetic Philosophy of Ancient Egypt and Greece.* Chicago: Yogi Publication Society Masonic Temple, 1912.

Wilson, Robert Anton. *Cosmic Trigger: Final Secret of the Illuminati.* Tempe, AZ: New Falcon, 1993.

bibliography

Achterberg, Jeanne. *Imagery in Healing: Shamanism and Modern Medicine.* Boston: Shambhala, 1985.

Beaulieu, John. *Music and Sound in the Healing Arts: An Energy Approach.* Barrytown, NY: Station Hill Press, 1987.

Becker, Robert O., and Gary Selden. *The Body Electric: Electromagnetism and the Foundation of Life.* New York: Morrow, 1985.

Bentov, Itzhak. *Stalking the Wild Pendulum: On the Mechanics of Consciousness.* Rochester, VT: Destiny Books, 1977.

Bonewits, Philip Emmons Isaac. *Real Magic: An Introductory Treatise on the Basic Principles of Yellow Magic.* Rev. ed. York Beach, ME: Weiser, 1989.

Castaneda, Carlos. *The Teachings of Don Juan: A Yaqui Way of Knowledge.* Berkeley, CA: University of California Press, 1968.

Chia, Mantak. *Awaken Healing Energy Through the Tao: The Taoist Secret of Circulating Internal Power.* New York: Aurora Press, 1983.

Crowley, Aleister. *Magick: Liber ABA Book Four,* 2nd rev. ed., ed. Hymenaeus Beta. York Beach, ME: Weiser Books, 1997.

DuQuette, Lon Milo. *Enochian Vision Magick: An Introduction and Practical Guide to the Magick of Dr. John Dee and Edward Kelley.* York Beach, ME: Weiser, 2008.

Eden, Donna, and David Feinstein. *Energy Medicine: Balance Your Body's Energies for Optimal Health, Joy, and Vitality.* New York: Jeremy P. Tarcher/Putnam, 1998.

Eliade, Mircea. *Shamanism: Archaic Techniques of Ecstacy.* Princeton, NJ: Princeton University Press, 1951.

Emoto, Masaru. *The Hidden Messages in Water.* Hillsboro, OR: Beyond Words, 2004.

Godwin, Joscelyn. *The Mystery of the Seven Vowels: In Theory and Practice.* Grand Rapids, MI: Phanes Press, 1991.

Goldman, Jonathan. *The Divine Name: The Sound That Can Change the World.* London: Hay House, 2010.

————. *Healing Sounds: The Power of Harmonics.* Rochester, VT: Healing Arts Press, 2002.

————. *Shifting Frequencies.* Flagstaff, AZ: Light Technology Publications, 1988.

Green, Elmer, and Alyce Green. *Beyond Biofeedback.* New York: Delacorte Press, 1977.

Haanel, Charles F. *The Master Key System.* S.l.: Filiquarian, 2006.

Hado USA. "Water Crystals Gallery." Accessed March 5, 2015. http://hadousa.com/gallery.html.

Halpern, Steven. "Healing Vibrations" in *Yoga Journal*, no. 114 (1994).

Harner, Michael J. *The Way of the Shaman.* 10th Anniversary Ed., 1st Harper ed. San Francisco: Harper, 1990.

Hart, Mickey, and Jay Stevens. *Drumming at the Edge of Magic: A Journey into the Spirit of Percussion.* San Francisco: Harper, 1990.

Henry, R. C. "The Mental Universe" in *NATURE* 436 (July 7, 2005).

Jenny, Hans. *Cymatics: A Study of Wave Phenomena and Vibration.* Newmarket, NH: MACROmedia, 2001.

Kalweit, Holger. *Shamans, Healers, and Medicine Men.* Boston: Shambhala, 1992.

Kenny, Robert. "The Science of Collective Consciousness," in *What Is Enlightenment: Redefining Spirituality for an Evolving World* (May 1, 2004).

Kraig, Donald Michael. *Modern Magick: Twelve Lessons in the High Magickal Arts.* Rev. ed. Woodbury, MN: Llewellyn Publications, 2010.

Lowitz, Leza, and Reema Datta. *Sacred Sanskrit Words: For Yoga, Chant, and Meditation.* Berkeley, CA: Stone Bridge, 2005.

Maharishi Programmes. "Maharishi Effect Research." Accessed February 14, 2015. http://maharishi -programmes.globalgoodnews.com/maharishi-effect /research.html.

Mathieu, W. A. *The Listening Book: Discovering Your Own Music.* Boston: Shambhala, 1991.

Mehrabian, Albert. *Silent Messages: Implicit Communication of Emotions and Attitudes.* Belmont, CA: Wadsworth, 1971.

Mumford, Jonn. *Magical Tattwas: A Complete System for Self-development.* St. Paul, MN: Llewellyn Publications, 1997.

Schafer, R. Murray. *The Soundscape: Our Sonic Environment and the Tuning of the World.* Rochester, VT: Destiny Books, 1993.

Tomatis, Alfred, and Billie Thompson. *The Conscious Ear: My Life of Transformation through Listening.* Barrytown, NY: Station Hill Press, 1991.

Touch the Sound: A Sound Journey with Evelyn Glennie, Directed by Thomas Riedelsheimer, 2004. New York: Filmquadrat, 2004, DVD.

Walla, Arjun. "The Illusion of Matter: Our Physical Material World Isn't Really Physical At All." Collective

Evolution. Accessed December 5, 2013. http://tinyurl.com
/kfcvykb.

Wilson, Robert Anton. *E-mail to the Universe: And Other Alterations of Consciousness.* Tempe, AZ: New Falcon, 2005.

Wilson, Tim. "Chant: The Healing Power of Voice and Ear," in *Music: Physician for Times to Come: An Anthology,* ed. Don Campbell. Wheaton, IL: Quest Books, 1991.

To Write to the Authors

If you wish to contact the authors or would like more information about this book, please write to the authors in care of Llewellyn Worldwide Ltd., and we will forward your request. Both the authors and publisher appreciate hearing from you and learning of your enjoyment of this book and how it has helped you. Llewellyn Worldwide Ltd. cannot guarantee that every letter written to the authors can be answered, but all will be forwarded. Please write to:

Joshua Goldman and Alec W. Sims
℅ Llewellyn Worldwide
2143 Wooddale Drive
Woodbury, MN 55125-2989

Please enclose a self-addressed stamped envelope for reply,
or $1.00 to cover costs. If outside the USA, enclose
an international postal reply coupon.

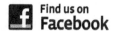